MW00674330

NUTRITION AND CANCER:

PRACTICAL TIPS AND TASTY RECIPES FOR SURVIVORS

By Sandra L. Luthringer, RD, LDN, and
Valerie J. Kogut, MA, RD, LDN

Pittsburgh, Pennsylvania

Hygeia Media, an imprint of the Oncology Nursing Society

ONS Publications Department
Interim Publisher and Director of Publications: Barbara Sigler, RN, MNEd
Managing Editor: Lisa M. George, BA
Technical Content Editor: Angela D. Klimaszewski, RN, MSN
Staff Editor II: Amy Nicoletti, BA
Copy Editor: Laura Pinchot, BA
Graphic Designer: Dany Sjoen

Library of Congress Cataloging-in-Publication Data
Luthringer, Sandra I.
    Nutrition and cancer : practical tips and tasty recipes for survivors / by Sandra L. Luthringer and Valerie J. Kogut.
      p. cm.
    ISBN 978-1-935864-02-8 (alk. paper)
    1. Cancer--Nutritional aspects. 2. Cancer--Diet therapy. I. Kogut, Valerie J. II. Title.
    RC268.45.L88 2011
    616.99'40654--dc22

                                                                                                2010046681

Publisher's Note

This book is published by the Oncology Nursing Society (ONS). ONS neither represents nor guarantees that the practices described herein will, if followed, ensure safe and effective patient care. The recommendations contained in this book reflect ONS's judgment regarding the state of general knowledge and practice in the field as of the date of publication. The recommendations may not be appropriate for use in all circumstances. Those who use this book should make their own determinations regarding specific safe and appropriate patient-care practices, taking into account the personnel, equipment, and practices available at the hospital or other facility at which they are located. The editors and publisher cannot be held responsible for any liability incurred as a consequence from the use or application of any of the contents of this book. Figures and tables are used as examples only. They are not meant to be all-inclusive, nor do they represent endorsement of any particular institution by ONS. Mention of specific products and opinions related to those products do not indicate or imply endorsement by ONS. Web sites mentioned are provided for information only; the hosts are responsible for their own content and availability. Unless otherwise indicated, dollar amounts reflect U.S. dollars.

ONS publications are originally published in English. Publishers wishing to translate ONS publications must contact ONS about licensing arrangements. ONS publications cannot be translated without obtaining written permission from ONS. (Individual tables and figures that are reprinted or adapted require additional permission from the original source.) Because translations from English may not always be accurate or precise, ONS disclaims any responsibility for inaccuracies in words or meaning that may occur as a result of the translation. Readers relying on precise information should check the original English version.

Printed in the United States of America

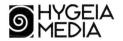

An imprint of the Oncology Nursing Society

Disclosure

Editors and authors of books and guidelines provided by the Oncology Nursing Society are expected to disclose to the readers any significant financial interest or other relationships with the manufacturer(s) of any commercial products.

A vested interest may be considered to exist if a contributor is affiliated with or has a financial interest in commercial organizations that may have a direct or indirect interest in the subject matter. A "financial interest" may include, but is not limited to, being a shareholder in the organization; being an employee of the commercial organization; serving on an organization's speakers bureau; or receiving research from the organization. An "affiliation" may be holding a position on an advisory board or some other role of benefit to the commercial organization. Vested interest statements appear in the front matter for each publication.

Contributors are expected to disclose any unlabeled or investigational use of products discussed in their content. This information is acknowledged solely for the information of the readers.

The contributors provided the following disclosure and vested interest information:

Valerie J. Kogut, MA, RD, LDN: honoraria, other remuneration, Nestlé Nutrition

CONTENTS

ACKNOWLEDGMENTS

The authors gratefully acknowledge the significant contributions of the following—both in content as well as their delicious recipes!

Sandra Boody, CDA, RDH, MEd, is a patient advocate, speaker for the National Cancer Institute Specialized Programs, head and neck cancer survivor, educator, and dental hygienist. She is a graduate of the University of Pittsburgh. Sandy has extensive teaching experience including nursing homes, vocational education, and community college and served as the director of a dental careers program for 26 years. She is currently an adjunct faculty member in the continuing education department in the School of Dental Medicine at the University of Pittsburgh. Her clinical experience includes hospitals, nursing homes, and private practice dentistry. She lectures extensively to patients as well as professionals on oral care for the patient with cancer.

Jacqueline Little is pursuing a Master of Science in Clinical Dietetics and Nutrition at the University of Pittsburgh. Jacqueline has worked in the food industry as a chef, weight management consultant, and sensory technician for the past 10 years. She operated her own personal chef and catering business in Los Angeles, California, servicing private clients for three years. She is currently interning at Giant Eagle's Corporate Headquarters in Pittsburgh, Pennsylvania, where she works in the Sensory and Nutrition Department. Jacqueline is passionate about food, cuisine, health, and nutrition; she is currently working on a cookbook and aspires to one day run her own wellness center.

Maria Q.B. Petzel, RD, CSO, LD, CNSC, is a senior clinical dietitian at the University of Texas MD Anderson Cancer Center in Houston. Maria received her Bachelor of Science degree in Nutritional Sciences from the University of Oklahoma Health Sciences Center in 2001. Since graduating, her focus has been on nutrition for patients with cancer. At MD Anderson, Maria received a joint appointment in the departments of Surgical Oncology and Clinical Nutrition, allowing her to specialize in the nutritional management of patients following major pancreatic and other gastrointestinal surgeries. She also holds specialty certifications in both oncology nutrition and nutrition support. Maria has authored several professional publications and is heading several clinical research projects. She has been honored as one of MD Anderson's Outstanding Patient Educators and was named as a Recognized Young Dietitian of the Year by the American Dietetic Association in 2008.

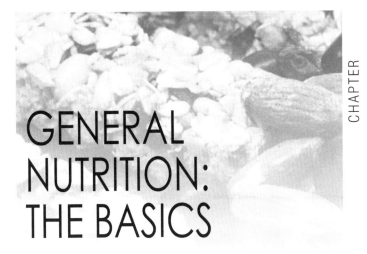

CHAPTER 1

GENERAL NUTRITION: THE BASICS

G ood nutrition is important for everyone. We are bombarded with information on diet and nutrition every day through the media. However, it is often not until we or someone we love is diagnosed with a serious illness like cancer that we stop cold in our tracks and take a long, hard look at our lifestyle, including what we eat. Some of the questions we may ask include

- "Did my diet in some way contribute to the diagnosis?"
- "Can I help treat my illness with dietary changes?"
- "Can my illness be cured by diet?"

Cancer is not simply one diagnosis with one treatment. There are many various types of cancers, and the treatments vary depending on the type and stage of cancer, general health and age of the patient, and the ultimate goals of the healthcare team and the patient. Just as the treatment plan varies from patient to patient, so do their nutritional needs. This book will provide some much-needed answers for the many questions you may have about diet and nutrition during this most stressful time.

THE BALANCED DIET

One of the most common questions asked of patients recently diagnosed with cancer is "Do I need to be on a special diet?" The answer is not so simple. There is no "one-size-fits-all" diet for patients with cancer. However, no matter what your nutritional needs are right now, it is never too late to adopt some healthy eating habits. Keep these important nutrition basics in mind as you plan your meals and snacks:

- **Balance is key.** Try to include foods from all food groups on most days. This includes grains, protein foods, fruits and vegetables, dairy, and even some fat.
- **Listen to your body.** Eat when you are hungry, and stop when you are satisfied. If cancer treatment has left you with little appetite, eat small amounts of food more often, such as every two to three hours.
- **Variety is vital.** Because food likes and dislikes change often, and especially during cancer treatment, adding variety to your diet can help you overcome this obstacle to maintaining good nutrition. Eating a variety of foods will help you get all the nutrients your body needs.
- **Make every bite count.** Increase your intake of whole grains, fruits, and vegetables when possible, and decrease the amount of sugar, fats, and "empty calories" you eat.

PUMP UP THE PROTEIN

Protein is an important nutrient to the healing process. Our bodies use protein to build tissues, blood cells, cells in the immune system, muscle, skin, and hair. Some illnesses such as cancer may increase our body's need for protein. Stress and injury also may increase our need for protein to help tissues heal and our bodies recover.

Ways to increase the protein in your diet:
- Include meat, fish, and poultry in your diet. If red meat is unappealing to you, experiment with fish or chicken or eat protein foods cold in salads, sandwiches, or spreads.
- Add dairy foods like milk, cheese, yogurt, pudding, or ice cream. Nonfat instant dry milk can even be added to milk, casseroles, soups, potatoes, or puddings for added protein without extra fat or flavor.
- Eggs are an excellent source of protein, and most patients can tolerate them well. Avoid raw or undercooked eggs, which may contain harmful bacteria.
- Peanut butter and hummus are great high-protein spreads for bread, crackers, fruits, and vegetables.
- Beans, legumes (like dried peas and beans), and tofu can be added to casseroles, pastas, soups, and spreads to add to your daily protein needs.

CHOOSE THE RIGHT FATS

All fats are bad, right? Wrong! We now know that there are good fats as well as bad fats, and we also know that fat plays an important role in a healthy diet. Fat is a good source of energy (in the form of calories) and provides flavor to foods. Food researchers now know that it is not necessarily the *amount* of fat in our diets but the *type* of fat that plays an important role in disease prevention. "Good" fats include unsaturated fats—those found in olive and canola oils, peanuts and other nuts, peanut butter, and avocados. These fats lower the level of total and "bad" LDL cholesterol, which accumulates in and clogs artery walls, while maintaining levels of "good" HDL cholesterol, which carries cholesterol from artery walls and delivers it to the liver for disposal. "Bad" fats include saturated fats—the heart-clogging kind found in butter, fatty red meats, and full-fat dairy products. "Very bad" fats are the manmade trans fats. These are the fats generally found in baked goods and prepackaged desserts and snacks.

Quick tips for choosing healthy fats:
- Use liquid plant oils for cooking and baking. Good choices for healthy fats include olive oil, canola oil, and other plant-based oils. These are rich in unsaturated fats—the "good" fats.
- Switch your spread from butter or stick margarine to soft tub margarine. Choose a product that has zero grams of trans fat and no hydrogenated oils. Canola or olive oil–based spreads are good choices.
- Ditch the trans fat. Trans fat is the "bad" fat and is found in most baked goods and processed snack foods.
- Go for the omega-3s. Foods like salmon, walnuts, almonds, and canola oil all provide good sources of omega-3 fatty acids, another "good" fat.
- Go lean on meat and milk. Meats and higher-fat dairy products are naturally high in saturated fats, so the leaner the better, and less fat is best. Buy lower-fat dairy products when possible, and always look for lean cuts of meat, avoiding highly processed luncheon meats that have added fat.

WATCH THE SUGAR

"Does sugar feed cancer?" This is a simple question without a simple answer. The bottom line is that sugar feeds *all* cells in the body. There is nothing special about cancer cells that makes them use the sugar that we eat more than any other cell in our bodies. Rest assured that even if you avoid all sugar in your diet, your body will find ways to make glucose to nourish your cells, generally out of protein and fat that has been stored in the body. Although sugar does not specifically target cancer cells for growth, a healthy diet should minimize the amount of sugar-containing foods. To reduce the amount of sugar you eat, follow these tips:

- High-sugar foods are generally high in calories and low in other nutrients. You may fill up on these foods, leaving no room for more nutritious foods that your body needs at this time. A healthy diet consists of high-quality foods like fruits, vegetables, protein foods, whole grains, and healthy fats.
- Eating high-sugar foods causes our bodies to produce more insulin. *Insulin* is a natural substance made by our bodies to encourage cell growth. For healthy cells, this is a good thing. However, some research suggests that excess insulin may encourage cancer cells to grow more, which is definitely not a good thing.
- Eating protein-containing foods, higher-fiber foods, and even foods with some fat will help your body process the sugar more slowly and will ultimately lower the amount of insulin produced. Yet another reason to eat a diet filled with healthier, more nutritious foods!
- Questions about artificial sweeteners and increased cancer risks have been posed since the early 1970s, when the use of saccharin was thought to cause an increase in bladder cancer in laboratory rats. Since then, however, results from further stud-

FOOD FOR THOUGHT:

"Red meat, coffee, and chocolate were three foods I simply could not tolerate during my cancer treatments, and I used to LOVE them all. I found that meats eaten cold, like thinly sliced roast beef from the deli, tasted so much better. And I guess giving up the bitter-tasting coffee and chocolate wouldn't hurt right now!"

—*Sally R., breast cancer survivor*

ies of this artificial sweetener, as well as all other approved sweeteners, have not demonstrated clear evidence of an association with cancer in humans. Because artificial sweeteners are many times sweeter than table sugar, smaller amounts are needed to create the same level of sweetness. When used in moderation, they can safely be part of a healthy diet plan.

Tips to help you find a healthy balance with your food choices:
- Stick with natural sugar found in foods like fruit. This is a much healthier option than the processed sugar that is found in candy, desserts, and baked goods.
- Avoid concentrated sources of sugar, such as sodas and fruit drinks. Drink 100% fruit juice in moderation, and avoid fruit drinks that don't contain any real fruit juice—and contain little nourishment.
- Practice moderation. Smaller portions eaten less often can easily fit into a healthy eating plan.
- Choose healthier options for snacks and treats, such as fruits, whole grain crackers and cereals, nuts, and seeds.

MODIFY YOUR DIET TO MANAGE SIDE EFFECTS

Although eating is a routine activity for most people, it can become anything but routine when you are not feeling well or are battling side effects from your cancer treatments. Just as there are many types of cancers and treatment options, people diagnosed with cancer all have differing degrees of nutritional needs. Nutritional modifications specific to the side effects of cancer and its treatment are individualized for each patient, and can change from time to time during the course of treatment. This book is a guide and reflects information contributed from healthcare professionals, caregivers, and patients just like you who have experienced some of the same nutritional issues.

RECIPES

ROASTED RED PEPPER HUMMUS

Protein is an important nutrient for those undergoing treatment for cancer. When protein foods like beef, poultry, or fish are no longer appealing, why not try hummus? It is a quick and easy high-protein dip that tastes great on crackers, rice cakes, or pita bread.

Ingredients

- 2 cloves garlic, minced
- 1 can (15 oz) garbanzo beans, drained
- ⅓ cup tahini (sesame paste)
- ⅓ cup lemon juice
- ½ cup roasted red peppers
- ¼ teaspoon dried basil

Directions

- In an electric food processor, combine garlic, garbanzo beans, tahini, and lemon juice.
- Process until smooth.
- Add roasted peppers and basil and blend until peppers are finely chopped.
- Season if desired with salt and pepper.
- Keep refrigerated and serve chilled.

Makes 4 servings

Nutrition Facts

Per ½-cup serving: 275 calories, 25 g fat, 12 g carbohydrates, 5 g fiber, 9 g protein, 490 mg sodium

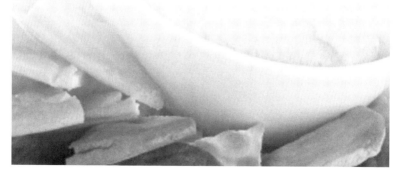

SNACK GRANOLA

The type of fat you eat may make a difference. Research shows that good fats like those found in nuts like walnuts, pecans, and almonds will provide you with not only some added protein but also some good omega-3 fatty acids. Keep this granola in a sealed airtight container, and add some to your salads, yogurt, or ice cream, or just eat it alone.

Ingredients

- 5 cups quick-cooking oats
- ½ cup wheat germ
- 1 cup non-fat dry milk
- 1 cup sesame seeds
- 2 cups dried fruit, such as raisins, cranberries, apricot, bananas, pineapple, or mango
- 1 cup flaked coconut
- ½ cup chopped walnuts or pecans
- ½ cup slivered almonds
- 1 cup canola oil
- 1 cup honey

Directions

- Preheat oven to 300°F.
- Combine all dry ingredients in a very large bowl and mix well.
- Warm the oil and honey on the stove or in the microwave and stir into the granola mixture.
- Spread mixture on cookie sheets and bake at 300° for 20 minutes, turning often until granola is a toasty brown.
- Allow to cool, then store in airtight containers.

Makes 20 servings

Nutrition Facts
Per ½-cup serving: 325 calories, 17 g fat, 39 g carbohydrates, 4 g fiber, 7 g protein, 31 mg sodium

BERRY APPLE CRISP

Keeping your diet low in simple sugars does not mean you have to give up great-tasting desserts! Try this fruit crisp for a delicious end to dinner, an evening snack, or anytime you need a little treat.

Ingredients

Filling

3 medium-sized baking apples, cored and thinly sliced
2 cups unsweetened frozen mixed berries

1 teaspoon cinnamon
2 tablespoons flour

Topping

1 cup quick-cooking oats
½ teaspoon cinnamon

¼ cup brown sugar
2 tablespoons butter or margarine

Directions

- Preheat oven to 325°F. Spray a 9-inch square metal or glass baking dish with nonstick cooking spray.
- Mix the apples, berries, cinnamon, and flour, and spoon into baking dish.
- In a small bowl, mix the topping ingredients until crumbly, and sprinkle over the fruit mixture.
- Bake at 325° for 30 minutes or until fruit is soft and topping is golden brown.

Makes 9 servings

Nutrition Facts

Per serving: 113 calories, 3 g fat, 18 g carbohydrates, 3 g fiber, 2 g protein, 31 mg sodium

TANGERINE MUFFINS

Many patients undergoing cancer therapy find tart foods much better toler-ated than sweet foods. These tasty muffins provide just the right amount of "pucker power" to satisfy your desire for tart!

Ingredients

- 1 cup all-purpose or whole wheat flour
- 1½ teaspoons baking powder
- 2 tablespoons sugar
- ¼ teaspoon salt
- ½ cup nonfat milk
- 1 egg white, slightly beaten
- 1 tablespoon canola oil
- 1 teaspoon vanilla extract
- ½ cup fresh tangerine sections, coarsely chopped

Directions

- Preheat oven to 400°F. Lightly coat mini muffin cups with nonstick cooking spray.
- In a medium bowl, stir together flour, baking powder, sugar, and salt. Set aside.
- In a small bowl, combine milk, egg white, oil, and vanilla.
- Add the egg mixture to the flour mixture, and stir just until moist-ened. The batter will be lumpy. Fold in the tangerine sections.
- Divide the batter into 18 mini muffin cups.
- Bake 14 minutes or until golden brown.

Makes 18 servings

Nutrition Facts

Per serving (1 muffin): 43 calories, 1 g fat, 8 g carbohydrates, 1 g fiber, 1 g protein, 59 mg sodium

CHAPTER 2

APPETITE CHANGES

People with cancer often experience chang-es in their appetite. This may be caused by changes in taste and smell, feeling full most times, or just being too tired to eat.

TASTE AND SMELL CHANGES

Why do some people have changes in taste and smell?

- The tumor itself can produce substances that result in taste changes.
- Chemotherapy drugs and biologic therapies such as interleukin-2 and interferon can alter the cells in the oral cavity.
- Radiation therapy: Depending on the location and dose of radiation, taste and smell changes may occur after two weeks of treatment and last for a few weeks after treatment. Some patients re-port taste and smell changes lasting for much lon-ger, up to a year, after the treatments are complet-ed.

- Bone marrow transplant: Recovery of taste buds usually occurs 45–60 days after transplantation.
- Medications such as antibiotics and pain medications can cause dry mouth and yeast infections in the mouth, which affect taste.

What can I do to deal with taste changes?

- Incorporate other protein foods in place of beef and pork, such as chicken or fish.
- Try food in various forms. If you can't tolerate an apple, try applesauce or apple juice.
- Experiment with different textures, temperatures, and seasonings.
- Salty foods may be preferred, such as pizza, sausage, chili, spaghetti sauce, and ketchup.
- Drink liquids such as water with lemon, tea, ginger ale, or fruit juices mixed with club soda to remove some of the strange tastes in your mouth. (Tart liquids like cranberry juice or lemonade seem to work better than sugary ones like soft drinks.)
- Use plastic utensils if foods taste like metal.
- Eat mints (or sugar-free mints), chew gum (or sugar-free gum), or chew ice to mask the bitter or metallic taste.
- Tart slushies or Italian ice works well too! Try lemon or raspberry ices—the more tart, the better.
- Rinse your mouth with cool black or green tea, lightly salted water, or baking soda and water. These liquids can "freshen" and cleanse your taste buds before eating.
- Do not eat canned food products if metallic taste is a problem.
- Experiment with eating cold foods like sandwiches, cottage cheese, and yogurt.

- Carry a bottle of salt water with you so you can swish and spit throughout the day.
- Eat starchy foods, such as bread, potatoes, rice, and plain pasta.
- Do not eat one to two hours before chemotherapy and up to three hours after therapy. It is common to develop a taste aversion to foods eaten during this time, so it is particularly important to avoid your favorite foods at this time.
- Use fruit-based marinades or honey glazes with vegetables and meats to help improve their flavor. Try chicken with a honey glaze or fish with lemons and oranges. You may be pleasantly surprised that adding fruit can drastically improve the flavor. Marinate the meat in a sweet or sour sauce.

FOOD FOR THOUGHT:

"I use sea salt to give food more flavor."

—*Dan P., bladder cancer survivor*

"I find that tart foods taste better to me than sweet, so I add extra calories with a cranberry smoothie instead of a milkshake."

—*Ruth E., colon cancer survivor and prior chemotherapy recipient*

What can I do if things smell bad?

- Cover beverages; try using a cup with a lid or drink through a straw.
- Select foods that do not need to be cooked, such as cheese, yogurt, peanut butter, and canned fruit.
- Have others prepare food so you can stay clear of the kitchen.
- Avoid foods with a strong aroma like fried chicken, fried fish, and foods from the cabbage family (including broccoli).

Emerging Research:
Research has shown that taking zinc sulfate during treatment may speed up the return of taste after radiation to the head and neck area.

Halyard, M.Y., Jatoi, A., Sloan, J.A., Bearden, J.D., Vora, S.A., Atherton, P.J., ... Loprinzi, C.L. (2007). Does zinc sulfate prevent therapy-induced taste alterations in head and neck cancer patients? Results of a phase III double-blind, placebo-controlled trial from the North Central Cancer Treatment Group (N01C4). *International Journal of Radiation Oncology, Biology, Physics, 67*, 1318–1322.

FEELING FULL

What is early satiety?

Early satiety is the feeling of being full after you have eaten a small amount, maybe only a few bites. This can sometimes be described as having a poor appetite.

What can cause early satiety?

Early satiety is a common side effect of chemotherapy or surgery. It can also be related to specific types of cancer, such as

- Gynecologic—fluid buildup from the tumor itself
- Lymphoma—abdominal mass or enlarged spleen
- Gastrointestinal—enlarged liver or cancer of the stomach
- Lung—difficulty breathing or shortness of breath
- Liver/pancreas—metabolic effects of the tumor.

What are the treatments for poor appetite/early satiety?

- Eat six small meals a day, making every bite count.
- Chew your food slowly.
- Avoid greasy foods and foods that are covered with high-fat sauces.

- Drink liquids 30 minutes before or after meals/ snacks instead of with your meals to keep from filling up on liquids.
- Drink only liquids of high nutritional value, avoiding water or other fluids without calories.
- Add milkshakes or liquid nutrition supplements to your diet.
- Avoid high-fiber and fatty foods that may fill you up and take longer for your body to digest.

- Try to consume one-third of your daily protein and calorie requirements at breakfast, generally the meal at which you are able to eat the most.
- Experiment with different foods eaten at different times of the day. Eat breakfast foods at dinnertime!
- Think of food as part of your treatment: Eat by the clock, every two hours like medicine.
- Have little dishes of nuts or trail mix near your computer or television or in your work area so you can grab a handful at any time and snack.

What are some foods that I should eat?

- Cheese and crackers
- Muffins
- Puddings
- Milkshakes or liquid nutrition supplements
- Yogurt
- Ice cream
- Energy/protein bars
- Powdered milk added to foods such as pudding, milkshakes, or any recipe using milk; using powdered milk in addition to liquid milk doubles the amount of nutrients in the food.
- Keep finger foods handy for snacking, such as deviled eggs, cream cheese or peanut butter on crackers or celery, deviled ham on crackers.

FATIGUE

What is cancer-related fatigue?

Cancer-related fatigue is one of the most common side effects of cancer and its treatment. Its exact cause is unknown, and it is not predictable by tumor type, treatment, or stage of illness. Usually, it comes on suddenly, does not result from activity or exertion, and is not relieved by rest or sleep. It is often described as "overwhelming." It may continue even after treatment is complete. Cancer-related fatigue could be made worse if you are not eating enough or you are not eating healthy foods.

What nutrition tips can help me to lessen fatigue?

- Drink plenty of fluids. Dehydration can worsen fatigue.
- Avoid eating sugary foods like candy, soft drinks, cakes, cookies, and pies. These foods might give a quick energy boost; however, this will wear off and you will be even more tired afterward.
- Try having some protein, fat, or fiber with each meal and snack. Protein, fat, and fiber can help keep blood sugar levels more stable. They will give you a prolonged feeling of energy from the food you eat.
- Use foods that are already prepared and just need to be heated for at least one meal a day.
- Try eating five or six small meals each day instead of three large ones.
- Eat well during "up" times— generally early in the morning.

FOOD FOR THOUGHT:
"I like to use foods that only need to be reheated, especially in the evening when I feel more tired and don't have the energy to cook."
—Tom W., lymphoma survivor

- Set a timer for 60-minute intervals. Eat a few bites and drink some fluids whenever the timer goes off.
- Eat a few bites every time a commercial comes on TV.

How can exercise help to decrease the effects of fatigue?

- You may feel too tired to exercise, but if you nap or just sit around, you will feel worse. Individuals with cancer who exercise a small amount each day feel better. Even small amounts of activity are better than none.
- Try taking a short (15–20-minute) walk each day.

What are other suggestions that can help to lessen the effects of fatigue?

- Use disposable paper plates, napkins, and cups. This cuts down on cleanup after meals.
- Ask family and friends to assist with shopping, cooking, and meal preparation. Plan this in advance for a few times a week.
- Get eight hours of sleep a night.

RECIPES

VEGGIE QUESADILLA WITH GREEK YOGURT, SALSA STYLE

Quesadillas are always quick, easy, and flavorful. You can use virtually any cheese, vegetable, and even leftover cooked chicken or cooked steak. The Greek yogurt salsa is a cooling addition to this dish.

Ingredients

- 2 teaspoons canola or olive oil
- 2 whole wheat tortillas, 8-inch size
- ½ cup shredded cheese—Try a cheddar and Monterey jack mix, crumbled feta, or your favorite nondairy cheese.
- 1 cup fresh spinach, chopped, or ½ cup diced cooked broccoli, zucchini, or green onion
- ½ cup diced red, yellow, or orange bell peppers, tomato, or red onion

Directions

- Heat a large skillet or electric griddle over medium heat. Coat with canola or olive oil.
- Place one tortilla on hot skillet or griddle. Sprinkle with shredded cheese and chopped vegetables, then top with remaining tortilla.
- Cook one side until crisp, about 3 minutes; flip carefully and cook for another 3 minutes.
- Remove from pan onto a cutting board, and cut into 4 pieces.
- Serve hot with Greek yogurt, salsa style (recipe follows).

Makes 2 servings

Nutrition Facts

Per serving: 355 calories, 20 g fat, 26 g carbohydrates, 3 g fiber, 6 g protein, 200 mg sodium

GREEK YOGURT, SALSA STYLE

This yogurt salsa is also tasty as a dip, dressing, or spread. Try it with tortilla chips, on chili, or with vegetables. It is high in protein and calcium.

Ingredients

½ cup plain nonfat Greek yogurt or strained plain yogurt

2 tablespoons diced tomato, seeds removed

1 tablespoon minced onion

¼ teaspoon garlic

⅛ teaspoon cumin

1 tablespoon chopped parsley or cilantro (optional)

Salt and pepper to taste

Directions

- Mix all ingredients in a small bowl. Adjust seasonings to taste.
- Cover with plastic wrap and refrigerate until ready to serve.

Makes 4 servings

Nutrition Facts

Per serving: 20 calories, 0 g fat, 3 g carbohydrates, 3 g fiber, 2 g protein, 15 mg sodium

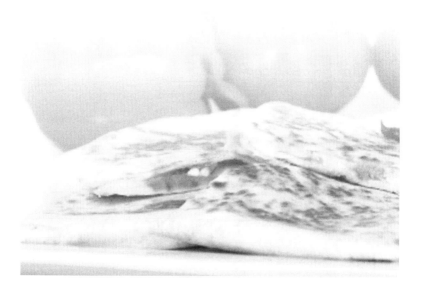

APPLE AND CHEDDAR QUESADILLA

Another great quesadilla idea! The sweetness of the apples and the saltiness of the cheese will surely tingle your taste buds. Experimenting with different foods is helpful when your appetite is not what it used to be.

Ingredients

- 2 teaspoons canola or olive oil
- 2 whole wheat tortillas, 8-inch size
- ½ cup shredded low-fat cheddar cheese; or try Monterey jack, brie, or other favorite cheeses
- One-half of an apple, thinly sliced; try granny smith, Fuji, or your favorite variety

Directions

- Heat a large skillet or electric griddle over medium heat. Coat with canola or olive oil.
- Place a tortilla on hot skillet or griddle. Layer with cheese and apples, then top with other tortilla.
- Cook one side until crisp, about 3 minutes; flip carefully and cook for another 3 minutes.
- Remove from pan onto a cutting board, and cut into 4 pieces.
- Serve hot. Try it with honey-mustard on the side.

Makes 2 servings

Nutrition Facts
Per serving: 361 calories, 20 g fat, 26 g carbohydrates, 3 g fiber, 10 g protein, 340 mg sodium

BROWN RICE SALAD WITH CORN AND SPINACH

This hearty salad with a tangy dressing will awaken your taste buds. The veggies can be cooked if needed or switched out for a frozen vegetable mix instead. Keeps for 4–5 days in the refrigerator. Can be frozen in individual baggies and reheated to serve as a warm side dish.

Ingredients

Salad

- 2 cups brown rice, cooked according to package directions
- 1 cup frozen white or sweet yellow corn, thawed and drained
- 2 cups fresh spinach, washed and chopped
- ½ cup sliced red onion
- 1 tomato, diced, or 3/4 cup cherry tomatoes, halved
- ⅓ cup dried cranberries, raisins, nuts or seeds, olives, low-fat feta, or other veggies (optional)

Dressing

4 tablespoons red wine vinegar
2 tablespoons olive or canola oil
½ teaspoon sugar
Salt and pepper to taste

Directions

- Whisk dressing ingredients together in a small bowl, and set aside.
- Toss all salad ingredients together in a large bowl. If preparing ahead of time, toss with dressing just before serving.

Makes 6 servings

Nutrition Facts

Per serving: 165 calories, 6 g fat, 25 g carbohydrates, 2.5 g fiber, 3 g protein, 231 mg sodium

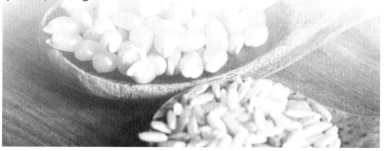

MIXED VEGETABLE STIR-FRY SERVED IN PITA WITH GREEK YOGURT

Vegetables are difficult to eat when you are not feeling well. This quick and easy recipe helps to get those vegetable servings into your diet. The vegetable mix is flavorful and can be made ahead of time; just heat as needed. The Greek yogurt adds protein, calcium, and a tangy topping.

Ingredients

2 tablespoons olive oil
1 onion, sliced
1 red pepper, sliced
1 green pepper, sliced
1 small zucchini, sliced

2 teaspoons minced fresh garlic
4 small whole wheat pita loaves
1 cup nonfat Greek yogurt
Salt and pepper to taste

Directions

- Slice whole wheat pitas in half.
- Season Greek yogurt to taste with your favorite herbs and spices.
- Heat a skillet to high heat and swirl olive oil in skillet. Carefully add vegetables and stir-fry, mixing often with wooden or silicone spoon until lightly cooked and browned. Season to taste.
- Fill pitas with vegetable mixture, and top with Greek yogurt.

Makes 4 servings

Nutrition Facts

Per serving: 185 calories, 6 g fat, 5 g protein, 35 g carbohydrates, 2.5 g fiber, 245 mg sodium

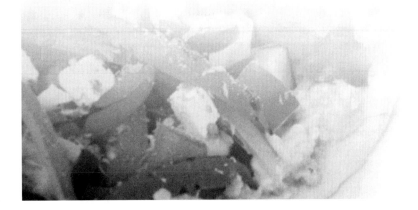

DARK COCOA AND DARK CHOCOLATE CHIP COOKIES

These cookies are a delicious way to awaken your taste buds. They are a good source of protein and antioxidants, and they keep well at room temperature. The cookie dough can be stored in the refrigerator and baked off a few at a time.

Ingredients

2 cups white whole wheat flour or all-purpose flour
½ cup vanilla soy or whey protein
½ cup dark cocoa powder
1 teaspoon salt
1 teaspoon baking soda
½ teaspoon baking powder

1 cup dark chocolate chips or chopped dark chocolate
1 cup brown sugar
¼ cup sugar
2 eggs
½ cup vanilla yogurt
2 teaspoons vanilla extract

Directions

- Preheat oven to 350°F. Spray a cookie sheet with nonstick cooking spray.
- Combine dry ingredients in a medium-size bowl.
- In a large bowl, beat sugar and eggs until smooth and fluffy, about 2 minutes. Add yogurt and vanilla and beat until mixed.
- Add the dry ingredients to the egg mixture, and stir to combine.
- Scoop dough with a tablespoon onto prepared cookie sheet. Flatten dough slightly.
- Bake for 11–13 minutes for soft cookies, 13–14 for crunchier cookies.
- Transfer cookies to rack and cool. Store in an airtight container.

Makes 30 servings

Nutrition Facts

Per cookie: 120 calories, 3 g fat, 5 g protein, 21 g carbohydrates, 2 g fiber, 113 mg sodium

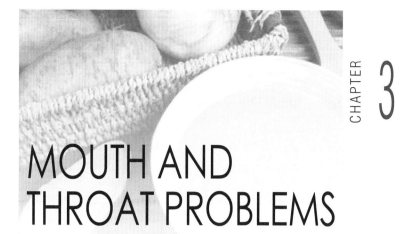

CHAPTER 3

MOUTH AND THROAT PROBLEMS

M outh and throat problems can be caused by a variety of different factors including the tumor itself, surgery, chemotherapy medications, and radiation therapy treatments. Some of these problems may occur only while you are undergoing cancer treatment, whereas other side effects may linger for weeks or even months after the treatment has finished. Mouth and throat problems may include difficulty chewing, dry mouth, difficulty swallowing, thick saliva, or sores in your mouth or throat.

DIFFICULTY CHEWING

Difficulty chewing can result from pain in the mouth, stiffness or pain in the jaw muscles, or problems with the teeth. Difficulty with chewing meats, fruits, and vegetables can make it hard to eat a nutritious diet. A person who wears dentures may temporarily be unable to use them for chewing because of pain or swelling in the mouth or gums.

What can cause difficulty when chewing?

- Soreness, pain, or inflammation in the mouth
- Dry mouth from radiation therapy to the mouth or neck region, chemotherapy, dehydration, or medications, including anti-nausea drugs, antidepressants, anti-anxiety medications, high blood pressure medications, and pain relievers. (More than 400 medications are known to cause dry mouth symptoms.)
- Gum disease, tooth decay, or tooth loss, which are possible long-term side effects of dry mouth, radiation therapy, or high-dose chemotherapy
- Infections of the mouth after radiation therapy or chemotherapy
- Pain and stiffness in the jaw muscles, either as a possible long-term side effect of radiation therapy or from jaw clenching or teeth grinding
- Mouth pain caused by nerve damage from some types of chemotherapy
- Tissue and bone loss in the jaw, a possible long-term side effect of radiation therapy to the mouth or jaw region
- Physical changes to the mouth, jaw, or tongue as a result of surgery

Diet and eating tips for patients with difficulty chewing

- Eat soft, smooth foods (such as cooked cereals, tofu, cottage cheese, mashed potatoes or sweet potatoes, yogurt, pudding, and ice cream).
- Mash or blend foods to make homemade shakes, or add blended vegetables or ground meats to casseroles or soups.
- Moisten dry foods with broth, sauces, butter, or milk.

- Take sips of water or other liquids while eating to keep the mouth and food moist.
- Try softer versions of your favorite fruits or vegetables, like applesauce or pureed carrots; switch to softer fruits and vegetables, such as bananas or peas; or consider eating commercially available meals made specifically for babies and toddlers.
- Cut food into small bites and chew slowly and thoroughly.

FOOD FOR THOUGHT:
"I find that if I drink more smoothies and milkshakes, it really helps me to get my calories and protein in and I don't have to worry about chewing anything. I am finding so many creative uses for my blender now that I have difficulty chewing since my dentures just don't fit right since the radiation therapy."

—*Lois, cancer survivor with prior radiation therapy to the tongue*

- If you are losing weight, eat smaller, more frequent meals that are high in protein and calories, such as eggs, milkshakes, casseroles, and nutritional shakes.

DIFFICULTY SWALLOWING

What is dysphagia?

Dysphagia, also known as difficulty swallowing, can occur because of the location of the tumor, the surgical site, or side effects of cancer treatment, such as radiation therapy to the neck and throat area.

What are the signs of difficulty swallowing?

- Coughing when eating
- Drooling
- Food being "pocketed" in your mouth
- Pain in throat or mid-chest when you swallow
- Feeling like the food is "sticking" on its way down
- Sensation of a lump in the throat

- Wheezing or breathing difficulty when eating
- Loss of appetite or weight loss
- Unexplained bouts of pneumonia or bronchitis
- Heartburn or indigestion
- Food or liquid forced up through the nose or throat
- Hoarseness or a "wet" or "gurgly" vocal quality after swallowing
- Throat clearing during meals

What can I do if I am having signs of dysphagia?

- Consider being evaluated by a speech and language pathologist, who can help you determine the appropriate food consistency that you can tolerate as well as provide you with some exercises to improve your swallowing function.
- Crush medicines that are in pill or tablet form; mix in juice, applesauce, jelly, or pudding. (Note: Check with your pharmacist first, as some medicines cannot be crushed or must be taken on an empty stomach.)
- If pain is a problem, use a numbing gel such as viscous lidocaine (by doctor's prescription) or over-the-counter liquid pain reliever such as acetaminophen oral suspension or ibuprofen suspension.
- Use a straw or a cup with a lid for liquids.
- Refrigerate food (the cold helps numb pain) or eat it cool or lukewarm. (Note: Pain in the esophagus may feel worse with cold liquids. If so, eat food at room temperature.)
- Eat bland foods that are soft and smooth but high in calories and protein (such as pudding, gelatin, ice cream, yogurt, and milkshakes).
- Eat small bites, and swallow each bite completely before taking another.

- Try thicker liquids (such as fruit that has been pureed in a blender) because they may be easier to swallow than thin liquids.
- Mash or blend foods to make homemade shakes, or moisten dry foods with broth, sauces, butter, or milk.
- Dunk breads in milk to make them soft.
- Try crushed ice in liquids at meals.
- Avoid alcohol and hot, spicy foods or liquids.
- Stay away from acidic foods, such as citrus fruits and drinks, and fizzy, carbonated drinks.
- Do not eat hard, dry foods such as crackers, nuts, potato chips, or seeds.
- Eat soft, moist foods like baked egg dishes, tuna salads, and casseroles.
- Avoid chewy foods or raw, crunchy vegetables and crusty breads.
- Add sauces and gravies to make meats easier to swallow.
- Maintain an upright position (as near $90°$ as possible) whenever eating or drinking, and remain in this position for 30–45 minutes afterward.
- Avoid talking while eating.
- If one side of the mouth is weak, place food into the stronger side of the mouth. At the end of the meal, check the inside of the cheek for any food that may have been pocketed.
- Try turning the head down, tucking the chin to the chest, and bending the body forward when swallowing. This often provides greater swallowing ease and helps prevent food from entering the airway.

FOOD FOR THOUGHT:

"I have found that the exercises that the speech therapist gave me to do really help me with my swallowing problem. Plus, I use lots of sauces and gravies on foods."

—*Leonard, head and neck cancer survivor and prior radiation therapy recipient*

- Do not mix solid foods and liquids in the same mouthful, and do not "wash foods down" with liquids unless you have been instructed to do so by your therapist. Instead, add moisture to the food. The two differing textures are confusing in the mouth, which can cause you to gag and choke.
- Eat in a relaxed atmosphere with no distractions.

THICK SALIVA

Radiation therapy to the head and neck areas, some types of chemotherapy, and certain other medicines can cause a thickening of the saliva. Dehydration may also contribute to thickened mucus.

What are some nutritional suggestions to help with thick saliva?

- Drink adequate amounts of fluid to prevent dehydration and help thin the saliva. If your intake is limited or weight loss is a concern, use calorie-containing fluids instead of noncaloric fluids like water, tea, and coffee. Aim for at least 48–64 ounces of fluid per day.

FOOD FOR THOUGHT:
"I carry my water bottle with me everywhere I go because the more fluid I can take in, the thinner my saliva is."
—Clyde, radiation therapy recipient

- Consume tart foods and beverages such as lemon-flavored soft drinks or soda water, sherbet, mandarin oranges, papaya, pineapple, sour lemon drops, bottled fruit-flavored beverages or iced teas, sports drinks, lemonade, orange-flavored drinks, or flavored ice pops. These may stimulate saliva secretion and thus thin the mucus.
- If milk products are found to increase mucus production, try low-fat dairy products or cooked items

(such as puddings or custards) before eliminating dairy products entirely. Soy-, rice-, or almond-based beverages may be better tolerated and can be used as a substitute for cow's milk.

- Drink clear liquid commercial nutrition supplements instead of milk-based shakes.
- Rinse your mouth frequently with club soda or a baking soda rinse (one-fourth teaspoon baking soda mixed in one cup water), especially before and after eating.
- Use tasty oils to lubricate the mouth before meals (such as olive, flaxseed, or sesame oil).
- Avoid beverages and foods containing caffeine (including soft drinks, black teas, coffees, and chocolate).

What other suggestions can help with thick saliva?
- Use a home humidifier.
- Mix one-half teaspoon of unseasoned meat tenderizer in one-half cup of water and rinse mouth with the solution. Do not swallow. The enzyme in meat tenderizers can assist in dissolving thick saliva.
- Use a straw. A straw may aid in hydration if nothing else and helps to push the fluid straight back to the throat so you can avoid trying to drink through the thick saliva.
- Use a non-alcohol-containing mouthwash.
- Take a water bottle with you every time you leave home.

SORE MOUTH OR THROAT

A sore mouth or throat can occur when cells inside your mouth, which grow and divide rapidly, are damaged by treatment such as bone marrow transplantation, chemotherapy, and radiation therapy to the mouth or throat area. These treatments may also affect rapidly dividing cells in the bone marrow, which may make you more susceptible to infection and bleeding in your mouth. Keeping your mouth clean promotes comfort and may prevent infection and improve nutrition.

What may cause a sore mouth?

- Certain chemotherapy drugs
- Radiation therapy to the mouth and neck
- Bone marrow transplantation therapy
- Poor nutrition

What should I do, and what should I look for?

- Have a dental evaluation and any problems corrected before starting treatment.
- Examine your mouth every day and look for redness, yellow or white patches, shininess, swelling, and sores or ulcerations in the mouth, gums, tongue, lips, or throat.
- Keep your mouth and teeth clean at all times. Brush your teeth with a soft-bristle toothbrush and nonabrasive fluoride toothpaste. Use only non-alcohol-containing mouth rinses.
- Remove bridges or dentures for cleaning after each meal and at bedtime.
- Tilt your head back and forth to help foods and liquid flow to the back of the throat for swallowing.
- Do not floss if your platelet count is low or if it causes pain or bleeding to the gums.
- Rinse your mouth or paint the irritated area with a swab dipped in a liquid antacid such as Maalox® or Mylanta®, or use a liquid numbing agent like prescription lidocaine.
- Avoid irritating spices, seasonings, and condiments such as pepper, chili powder, cloves, nutmeg, salsa, pepper sauces, and horseradish.

- Avoid rough foods such as dry toast, pretzels, and granola. They can be irritating to a sore mouth.
- Avoid citrus and acidic foods and beverages, fizzy drinks, high-sugar foods, or highly salted foods.
- Eat flavored ice pops or slushies, which can be very refreshing if you have a sore mouth or throat.
- Make ice chips using Enlive® or Resource Breeze® clear liquid nutritional supplements.
- Drink nectars such as peach, apricot, or guava.
- Eat well-cooked vegetables and canned fruit. Raw ones may hurt your mouth. You can also put fruits and vegetables through a blender.
- Avoid alcohol and tobacco.

FOOD FOR THOUGHT:
"My dietitian gave me a great idea that I found works well for me: I make ice chips out of clear liquids, especially those clear high-protein nutritional supplements. It helps me to get in some extra calories, and the cold feels good on my sore mouth.

—*Jenna, bone marrow transplant recipient*

Emerging Research:
Low-dose oral glutamine supplementation (10 g dissolved in liquid as a swish and swallow) during and after chemotherapy has been shown to significantly reduce both the duration and severity of chemotherapy-associated mouth sores. Oral glutamine appears to be a simple and useful measure to increase the comfort of many patients at high risk for developing mouth sores as a consequence of intensive cancer chemotherapy. You may want to consider asking your health-care provider how glutamine swish and swallow can benefit you if you have mouth sores.

Anderson, P.M., Schroeder, G., & Skubitz, K.M. (1998). Oral glutamine reduces the duration and severity of stomatitis after cytotoxic cancer chemotherapy. *Cancer, 83,* 1433–1439.
Peterson, D.E. (2006). New strategies for management of oral mucositis in cancer patients. *Journal of Supportive Oncology, 4*(2, Suppl. 1), 9–13.

DRY MOUTH

What causes a dry mouth?

- Medications
- Chemotherapy drugs
- Radiation treatment to the head and neck region

What are some ways to overcome a dry mouth?

- Use a water spray bottle to wet your mouth. Keep it near the places you work, sit, and sleep.
- Practice good oral hygiene.
- Use saliva substitutes such as the new line of MedActive® oral products that includes oral moisturizers (Patient-Friendly™ Oral Relief Rinse), lubricating sprays, moisturizing gels and lozenges (Oral Relief Lozenges, which come in lemon-lime, ruby raspberry, and orange crème flavors); MouthKote® spray; carboxymethyl or hydroxyethylcellulose solutions; Entertainer's Secret® spray; Glandosane® spray; or Moi-Stir® spray.
- Use a humidifier at night. Humidifiers add moisture to the air and can help decrease dry mouth during the night. Clean the humidifier regularly to prevent mold and bacteria buildup.
- Lubricate your lips with a moisturizing lip balm before going to sleep.
- Add a moisturizing saliva-enhancement gel or paste to tongue and gums at bedtime.
- Ask your dental professional to fabricate a soft night guard splint, and add oral moisturizing gel to the inside of the splint and wear it to sleep.
- Keep a glass of water on your nightstand. If dry mouth wakes you up, sipping on water may help wet your mouth during the night.

- Change your sleep routine. If you sleep with your mouth open or snore, try sleeping on your side to lessen the snoring. A sleep specialist may also help with other suggestions.
- Add gravies, sauces, and butter to your meals.
- Suck on—*do not chew*—ice or sugar-free flavored ice pops.
- Eat tart foods if you don't have sores in your mouth.
- Think cool: Eat soft-cooked chicken or fish that is room temperature; try thinned cereals (such as oatmeal made with plenty of water or milk that has been left to cool down); go for lukewarm (not scalding hot) soups and stews.

FOOD FOR THOUGHT:
"Sipping warm chicken stock from a mug between bites when eating a meal is both lubricating and nutritional. Ask friends who want to help to make homemade stocks, and freeze them in one-cup containers."

—*David J., larynx cancer survivor and prior radiation therapy recipient*

- Use a little olive, canola, avocado, or almond oil or yogurt, juice, jelly, or jam to make foods slippery and easier to swallow.
- Avoid sugary or acidic foods and candies because they increase the risk of tooth decay.
- Chew sugar-free gum with xylitol, and suck on sugar-free lozenges or hard candy.
- Add water-intensive fruits and vegetables such as melons (92% water), zucchini, and mushrooms to recipes.

What foods should I avoid if I have a dry mouth?

- Dry meats like beef, poultry, or pork without sauce or gravy
- Dry bread or rolls
- Pretzels
- Crackers
- Chips
- Cookies
- Cakes
- Dried fruit
- Peanut butter
- Nuts
- Popcorn
- Raw vegetables
- Coffee (even decaf)
- Caffeine

RECIPES

SQUASH, SWEET POTATO, AND GARLIC SOUP

Roasted squash makes an excellent soup; the carotenes in squash are better absorbed if prepared and eaten with a bit of oil.

Ingredients

1 acorn squash	4 cups chicken or vegetable
1 large sweet potato	stock
4 shallots (or 1 small onion)	½ cup low-fat sour cream or
5 medium cloves of garlic	Greek yogurt
2 tablespoons olive oil	Snip of chives or parsley

Directions

- Preheat oven to 350°F.
- Wash and scrub squash and sweet potato; cut in half and remove seeds from squash.
- Cut shallots in half, and coat squash, potato, shallots, and garlic cloves in oil. Place cut side of vegetables down in a shallow roasting pan and roast for 40–45 minutes until tender.
- Cool roasted vegetables and scoop out flesh; add to a stock pot with chicken or vegetable stock and bring to a boil.
- Simmer for 20–30 minutes, stirring occasionally until all vegetables are soft. Process the vegetables in a food processor and return to the stock pot; simmer until heated through. Ladle into soup bowls and garnish with a dollop of sour cream or yogurt and chives.

Makes 4 servings

Nutrition Facts
Per serving: 227 calories, 10 g fat, 3 g protein, 32 g carbohydrates, 4 g fiber, 310 mg sodium

CREAM OF BROCCOLI SOUP

A smooth and creamy way to add some nourishing veggies to your diet.

Ingredients

1 bunch fresh broccoli, chopped, or 2 (10 oz) packages frozen chopped broccoli

3 cups chicken stock

½ medium onion, chopped

4 tablespoons butter

5 tablespoons flour

1 pint half-and-half

Salt and white pepper to taste

Paprika, croutons, and parsley for garnish

Directions

- Cook broccoli and onion in stock until soft, about 10 minutes. Place in a blender and blend quickly, leaving some small pieces of broccoli out if desired.
- Using butter and flour, make a roux by cooking them in medium pot until it forms a paste.
- Add cream slowly, and stir constantly to prevent lumps.
- Mix in broccoli mixture. Add salt and pepper to taste, and garnish as desired. Serve hot or cold.

Makes 4 servings

Nutrition Facts

Per serving: 261 calories, 22 g fat, 5 g protein, 8 g carbohydrates, 3 g fiber, 200 mg sodium

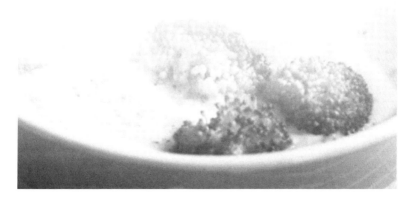

BREAKFAST VANILLA PUDDING

A sweet, tasty treat for breakfast, a snack, or even dessert. Experiment with your favorite nuts and dried fruits if desired, but it is delicious plain. Keep refrigerated until ready to serve. Warm in microwave if desired.

Ingredients

2 cups cold soy milk or whole milk

1 box instant vanilla pudding mix

½ cup vanilla protein powder

½ cup chopped almonds and ½ cup dried cranberries (optional)

Directions

- In a blender, combine milk, pudding mix, and protein powder and blend until smooth and thickened, about 1–2 minutes.
- Divide mixture among 4 small bowls. Sprinkle with almonds and cranberries, if desired.
- Chill until ready to serve.

Makes 4 servings

_____

Nutrition Facts
Per serving: 290 calories, 12 g fat, 7 g protein, 44 g carbohydrates, 3 g fiber, 420 mg sodium

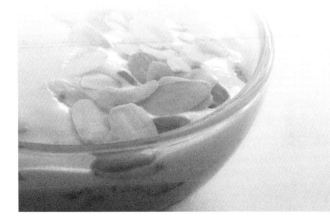

PROTEIN POWER PANCAKES

Pancakes with an extra protein boost! Add in blueberries, chopped apples, or chocolate chips. These can be made ahead of time and kept frozen until ready to serve. Top with maple syrup or strawberry sauce.

Ingredients

1 cup pancake mix
½ cup vanilla protein powder
1 cup water, whole milk, or soy milk

1 egg
1 tablespoon canola oil (reserve 1 teaspoon for griddle)

Directions

- Whisk ingredients together in a medium bowl until mixed thoroughly.
- Heat skillet or griddle on medium heat with 1 teaspoon of oil.
- Place ¼ cup of pancake mix on hot skillet, and cook for about 2 minutes on each side, flipping pancakes carefully once bubbles have formed on the top side. Cook until lightly browned.
- Serve warm with your favorite toppings.

Makes 4 servings

Nutrition Facts

Per serving: 180 calories, 6 g fat, 6 g protein, 24 g carbohydrates, 1.5 g fiber, 411 mg sodium

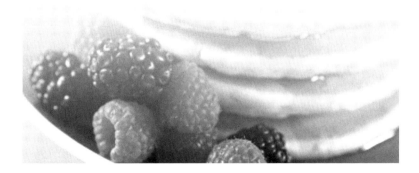

CHOCOLATE CHIP BREAD PUDDING

This recipe is great for breakfast, a snack, or even dessert. It has a soft, velvety texture and it can be made ahead of time and kept in the refrigerator for about five days. It can also be frozen; for an easy meal or snack, cut into portions and freeze in individual baggies. Reheat in microwave and top with maple syrup, caramel sauce, fruit, or ice cream!

Ingredients

10 slices of bread, cubed or torn into small pieces
4 eggs
1 cup sugar

1 cup milk, soy milk, or non-dairy creamer
2 teaspoons vanilla extract
½ cup chocolate chips

Directions

- Preheat oven to 350°F.
- Spray a 9" × 13" baking pan with cooking spray, and add bread cubes.
- In a bowl, whisk together eggs, sugar, milk or creamer, and vanilla.
- Pour mixture over bread cubes, and sprinkle with chocolate chips.
- Bake covered with foil for 35–45 minutes or until cooked through and internal temperature is 165°F.
- Remove from oven and allow to rest for about 10 minutes. Serve warm.

Makes 6 servings

_____

Nutrition Facts

Per serving: 450 calories, 10 g fat, 10 g protein, 68 g carbohydrates, 2 g fiber, 412 mg sodium

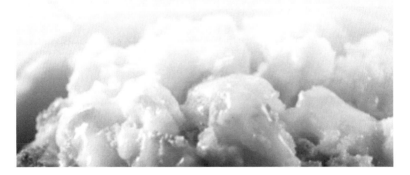

CHAPTER 4

GASTROINTESTINAL PROBLEMS

Not all patients with cancer will experience the eating and gastrointestinal-related side effects discussed in this chapter. However, you should know that there are many approaches to effectively deal with the basic challenges of eating and digesting food during treatment. As your symptoms change throughout the course of therapy, you can refer to the specific sections within this chapter for some guidance and support.

NAUSEA AND VOMITING

What is nausea?

Nausea is stomach distress with distaste for food and an urge to vomit.

What is vomiting?

Vomiting or *emesis* means throwing up. You may feel yourself breathing faster, you may feel dizzy, your heart may beat faster, and your skin may feel cool and clammy when you are about to vomit.

What are possible causes of nausea and vomiting?

- Nausea and vomiting can happen for many reasons. In people with cancer, it is most often the result of one or more medications, which interfere with the vomiting center in the brain.
- Chemotherapy or radiation therapy, which destroy tumor cells but in turn release chemicals that are irritating to your stomach
- Blockage in the stomach or intestines
- Certain tastes or smells, worry, and anxiety
- Treatment related to bone marrow and stem cell transplantation

What foods should I avoid?

- Fatty or greasy foods such as deep-fried foods, butter, oils, cheese, and cream sauces
- High-fat meats like bacon and sausage, which are hard to digest and are more likely to upset your stomach
- Spicy foods such as spaghetti, pizza, or tacos

What can I do to help prevent nausea or vomiting?

- Avoid smells or sights that can make you feel nauseated.
- Sit up or rest with your head and chest on pillows for one to two hours after eating.
- Rinse your mouth with mild salt water before and after meals to help alleviate the sour taste that may linger.
- Suck on peppermint or lemon candy if there is a bad taste in your mouth.
- Avoid eating for several hours prior to chemotherapy. If "dry heaves" are a problem, eat something

light and starchy, such as crackers, noodles, or dry toast, before your chemotherapy starts.

What should I do if I feel nauseated?

- Snack on dry foods such as toast, bagels, crackers, and pretzels.
- Do not eat large meals; eat several small meals instead.
- If you feel nauseated first thing in the morning, keep some crackers by your bed and eat them when you wake up.
- Avoid unpleasant odors; ask people to not smoke or wear heavy perfume around you.
- Eat slowly and in a peaceful environment.
- Distract yourself when eating alone; consider reading, watching television, or listening to music you love.
- Try low-odor, quick-preparation foods such as oatmeal, cream of wheat, cold cereal, canned fruit, shakes and smoothies, scrambled eggs, French toast, and pancakes.
- Experiment with food temperatures. Try warm foods such as oatmeal, cream of wheat, or soup and cold foods such as frozen fruit, flavored ice pops, frozen fruit bars, or shakes and smoothies. You'll quickly figure out what temperature your body likes best and when.
- Try unusual flavors. What you normally like may not be appealing now, and what you typically don't enjoy might actually work well during treatment. For example, try making a sweet shake or smoothie more tart by adding frozen cranberries into the mix.
- You can cut the overly sweet taste of liquid nutritional supplements by adding one or two teaspoons of

finely ground decaffeinated coffee to chocolate or vanilla flavors.

- Use a travel mug with a lid or straw to avoid unnecessary beverage aromas that can worsen nausea.
- Because hunger may last only a few minutes, keep snacks handy and eat the minute you feel hungry.
- Try keeping a little food in your stomach at all times. Having a completely empty stomach may worsen nausea.
- Sip ginger tea or ginger ale or suck on ginger candy between meals and snacks, as ginger has been shown to naturally reduce nausea.
- Drink plenty of fluids. Keeping hydrated can help a great deal with nausea. If you cannot do so on your own, your doctor may suggest fluid infusions.
- Ask your doctor or healthcare provider about medicines to help control nausea.

FOOD FOR THOUGHT:

"I have a fabulous neighbor. She cooks all of my food in her kitchen and then brings it to me all ready to eat. I find that I can eat a little better if I don't have to smell the food cooking, which makes me nauseous."

—*Shirley, lung cancer survivor receiving chemotherapy*

What can I do if vomiting has occurred?

- Do not drink or eat until you have the vomiting under control, then begin with sips of liquids.
- Keep track of how often and how much you are vomiting.
- Rinse out your mouth after vomiting to remove the sour taste.
- Take anti-nausea medication 30 minutes before eating.
- Carbonated beverages may help. Citrus-flavored soft drinks and ginger ale are usually easiest to tolerate.

DEHYDRATION

What is dehydration?

Dehydration is not having enough water in the body or not having enough fluid where it is needed in the body.

What are the signs of dehydration?

- Dry mouth and thirst
- Dizziness and weakness
- Constipation
- Having trouble swallowing dry food
- Dry or sticky tissues in the mouth that make it hard to talk
- Dry skin or skin that "tents" (stays up) when lightly pinched
- A swollen, cracked, or dry tongue
- Fever
- Weight loss
- Little or no urine or dark yellow-colored urine
- Fatigue

What can I do to prevent dehydration?

- Drink fluids.
- Remember that food contains fluid, too! Try to eat fruits, vegetables, soups, gelatins, and other moist foods. They contain up to 95% water!
- Avoid sugar and sugar-containing drinks. Sugar causes fluid to stay in the stomach longer. Soft drinks and most fruit drinks are high in sugar and should be diluted with water.
- Avoid foods high in sodium, as this will cause an increased need for even more fluid.

FOOD FOR THOUGHT:

"I take slices of fresh fruit like peaches, berries, and grapes and place them in ice cube trays. I use the fruit ice cubes to flavor water."

—*Barb R., breast cancer survivor*

"I put clear juice-type nutritional supplements like Resource® Breeze or Enlive® in ice cube trays and make ice chips, which then gives me extra calories as well as helps to keep me hydrated."

—*Lynn F., colon cancer survivor and chemotherapy recipient*

- Try to eliminate the cause of dehydration, such as vomiting, diarrhea, or fever.
- Apply lubricant to lips to avoid painful cracking.
- Keep a cooler filled with a variety of fluids like juices near your bed or chair, or fill a water bottle and keep it close by. Take sips often!
- Use ice chips to relieve dry mouth if you can't drink enough liquid.

DIARRHEA

What is diarrhea?

Diarrhea is the frequent passage of extremely soft or liquid stools.

What causes diarrhea?

Diarrhea may be caused by food reactions or the inability to digest milk and milk products. An emotional upset or infection may also be the cause. Some types of cancer treatments, such as chemotherapy, radiation therapy to the stomach and intestines, and bone marrow transplantation, may also cause diarrhea.

What types of foods may cause diarrhea?

- High-fat foods, such as processed meats, deep-fried foods, and chocolate
- Vegetables, especially uncooked vegetables and those of the cabbage family, spinach, corn, onions, and garlic
- Hard-to-digest high-fiber foods like nuts and seeds
- Dried beans and peas

What eating habits may help to control diarrhea?

- Follow a low-fiber, low-fat diet.

- Eat small, frequent meals.
- Do not eat hot or spicy foods.
- Drink liquids between—not with—meals.
- Avoid milk or milk products if they seem to make diarrhea worse.
- Avoid high-sugar foods, greasy foods, bran, raw fruits and vegetables, and caffeine.
- When the diarrhea starts to improve, try eating small amounts of foods that are easy to digest, such as rice, bananas, applesauce, yogurt, mashed potatoes, low-fat cottage cheese, and dry toast. If the diarrhea keeps getting better after a day or two, start eating small regular meals.

FOOD FOR THOUGHT:
"I go back to an old remedy that my pediatrician told me about for my kids. When I have diarrhea, I follow the BRAT diet: bananas, rice, applesauce, and toast."

—*Sophie K., ovarian cancer survivor receiving chemotherapy*

What types of foods are low in fiber?

- Soda crackers
- Gelatin
- Pasta
- Chicken noodle soup
- Some fruits, including bananas, watermelon, apricots, cantaloupe, honeydew, nectarines, papaya, and peaches (without the skin)
- White bread and refined cereals and rice products
- Canned or cooked fruits and vegetables
- Juices without pulp
- Tender, ground, or well-cooked meats

Emerging Research:
Probiotics have been shown to help manage diarrhea related to chemotherapy and radiation therapy. More research is still needed to determine the appropriate amounts and types to be used. If you

are experiencing diarrhea, discuss the use of probiotics with your healthcare professional. Some examples of probiotics include yogurt and Culturelle®.

Abd El-Atti, S., Wasieck, K., Mark, S., & Hegazi, R. (2009). Use of probiotics in the management of chemotherapy-induced diarrhea: A case study. *Journal of Parenteral and Enteral Nutrition, 33,* 569–570.

Fuccio, L., Guido, A., Eusebi, L.H., Grilli, D., & Cennamo, V. (2009). Effects of probiotics for the prevention and treatment of radiation-induced diarrhea. *Journal of Clinical Gastroenterology, 43,* 506–513.

CONSTIPATION

What is constipation?

Constipation is the irregular or difficult passage of hard stool, which often causes pain and discomfort.

What causes constipation?

Constipation can be caused by lack of activity, inadequate liquid intake, or not eating a variety of foods. Also, some types of medical treatment, pain medications, and chemotherapy drugs can cause constipation.

What should I look for?

- Stomach pains or cramps
- Belly appears expanded or puffy
- Vomiting or nausea
- Feeling of fullness or discomfort
- Changes in bowel habits, such as
  - Small, hard bowel movements
  - Seepage of soft stool resembling diarrhea
  - Passing an excess amount of gas or belching frequently
  - Absence of regular bowel movement within the previous three days

What should I do?

- Slowly increase the amount of high-fiber foods in your daily diet.
- Drink plenty of fluids (8–10 glasses per day). Try to drink highly nutritious fluids (such as milkshakes, eggnogs, and juices, as opposed to water) because liquids can be filling and reduce your appetite. Apple juice and prune juice may be particularly helpful, especially if heated.
- Increase physical activity, such as walking, as tolerated.
- Use laxatives and stool softeners as instructed by your doctor or healthcare provider.
- Use high-liquid foods, such as flavored ice pops, fruit, and soup, to get more fluid into your diet.
- Snack on fiber-rich dried fruit, such as apricots, raisins, dried plums (prunes), and dates.
- Eat a breakfast that includes a warm drink and fiber-rich foods, such as high-fiber cereal, oatmeal, and whole grain toast.
- If you have a lot of gas, avoid carbonated drinks, broccoli, cabbage, cauliflower, dried beans, peas, onions, brussels sprouts, Swiss chard, radishes, turnips, and watercress, all of which can worsen symptoms.

FOOD FOR THOUGHT:

"Whenever I feel constipated, I put some Kellogg's® All Bran® buds on my yogurt, and it really helps to relieve the problem."

—*Mary W., endometrial cancer survivor*

- Avoid drinking through straws and chewing gum, which can cause you to swallow air and feel even more bloated.
- Mix together three parts wheat bran cereal, two parts applesauce, and one part prune juice; eat this three times a day or more. Try this mixture on toast, or eat one tablespoon of it with your medications.

What foods are high in fiber?

- Whole wheat breads
- Whole grain cereals, such as oatmeal or bran cereal
- Fresh fruits and vegetables
- Dried fruits like raisins and prunes
- Bran, legumes, and flaxseed

What shouldn't I do?

- Do not strain or use extreme force in trying to move your bowels.
- Do not eat raw fruits or vegetables if your neutrophil count is less than $1,000/\text{mm}^3$.

RECIPES

GINGER-SCENTED CHILLED MELON SOUP

Ginger has been shown to be helpful in reducing nausea and helping with digestion. Try this cold soup prior to or between meals to help ease your stomach and improve your appetite.

Ingredients

4 cups ripe honeydew melon, cut into large chunks
1¼ teaspoons fresh ginger, finely chopped
4 tablespoons fresh lime juice
2 tablespoons scallions, sliced, plus more for garnish
¾ cup apple juice
½ teaspoon kosher salt
1 cup English cucumber, un-peeled and diced
2 tablespoons finely chopped cilantro or mint
4 teaspoons light sour cream, for garnish

Directions

- In a blender, combine melon chunks, ginger, lime juice, scallions, apple juice, and salt. Blend until smooth and creamy.
- Refrigerate the soup until chilled, about 30 minutes.
- Divide soup among four small bowls or glasses. Garnish with diced cucumber and cilantro or mint and a dollop of light sour cream.

Makes 4 servings

Nutrition Facts

Per serving: 97 calories, 1 g fat, 1 g protein, 21 g carbohydrates, 2 g fiber, 300 mg sodium

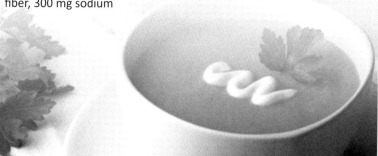

GINGER TEA INFUSION WITH FRESH MINT

This refreshing drink will aid gastrointestinal problems.

Ingredients

4–5 fresh mint leaves
  2 tablespoons agave nectar or
    honey (optional)

1–2-inch piece of fresh ginger,
  washed
4 cups water

Directions

- Cut unpeeled ginger into small pieces.
- In a medium pot, bring ginger and water to a boil. Reduce heat and simmer for 10 minutes, covered.
- Sweeten with agave nectar or honey, if desired. Add fresh mint; cover and allow to infuse for 10 minutes.
- Strain into a pitcher using a fine colander. Serve warm or iced.

Makes 4 servings

Nutrition Facts

Per 1 cup sweetened serving: 30 calories, 0 g fat, 0 g protein, 8 g carbo-hydrates, 0 g fiber, 20 mg sodium

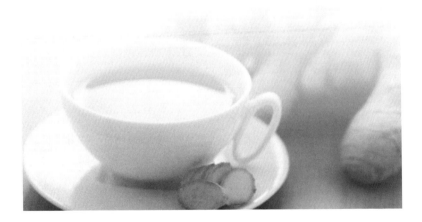

EASY MAPLE-SPICED APRICOT RICE PUDDING

Comfort food at its best. This easy-to-make meal will tingle your taste buds and keeps well in the refrigerator. It's light and a little sweet, so it's easy to eat when you're not feeling well. The ginger aids nausea too, so use more if you like. Just warm in the microwave or enjoy chilled.

Ingredients

- 1 cup instant rice
- 3 cups almond milk or soy milk
- ⅓ cup dried apricots, cut into quarters
- ¼ cup maple syrup

- ½ teaspoon salt
- ½ teaspoon ground cinnamon or 1 stick cinnamon
- ¼ teaspoon ground ginger

Directions

- Combine ingredients in a medium saucepan.
- Bring to a boil and then reduce heat to a simmer, stirring occasionally.
- Cook for about 5 minutes or until rice has absorbed liquid.
- Remove from heat and let sit covered for 15–20 minutes. Serve warm.

Makes 4 servings

Nutrition Facts

Per serving: 197 calories, 2.5 g fat, 3 g protein, 40 g carbohydrates, 2 g fiber, 10 mg sodium

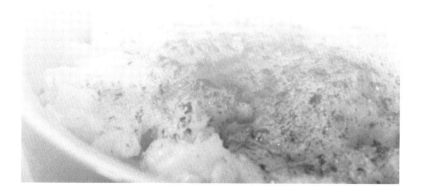

WHOLE GRAIN APPLE BARS WITH MILLET

These bars are fun to make and are a healthy treat. They are rich in whole grains, a good source of fiber, and super tasty. They keep well refrigerated or frozen, and make a lovely snack, treat, or quick breakfast.

Ingredients

Crust and Topping

- ½ cup whole wheat flour
- ½ cup all-purpose flour
- ¾ cup old-fashioned oats
- ¼ cup flaxseed meal
- 3 tablespoons millet, raw
- 1 teaspoon baking powder
- ¼ teaspoon salt
- 1 teaspoon cinnamon
- ½ cup brown sugar
- 2 egg whites, beaten with 2 tablespoons nonfat plain yogurt

Filling

- 3 cups baking apples (about 3 medium apples)
- ¼ cup orange or apple juice
- 2 tablespoons light brown sugar
- 2 tablespoons all-purpose flour

Directions

- Preheat oven to 375°F. Spray a 9" × 7" baking dish with nonstick spray.
- In a medium bowl, combine crust and topping ingredients, mixing until combined. The mixture should be crumbly.
- Press ¾ of the mixture onto the prepared baking pan. Bake for 8 minutes; remove from oven and set aside.
- While crust is baking, peel and dice apples and toss with juice, sugar, and flour.
- Top baked crust with diced apple mixture and the rest of the topping mixture.
- Bake for 30–32 minutes. Remove to rack and allow to cool.
- Cut into 12 squares. Serve for breakfast, snack, or dessert.

Makes 12 servings

Nutrition Facts

Per serving: 194 calories, 3 g fat, 5 g protein, 36 g carbohydrates, 2.5 g fiber, 60 mg sodium

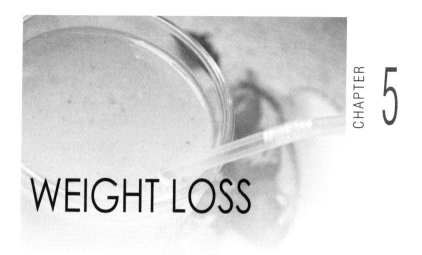

CHAPTER 5

WEIGHT LOSS

Often, patients with cancer are not able to take in adequate amounts of calories and protein. These are essential during the recovery process to help your body heal as well as to tolerate the treatments better.

ADDING MORE CALORIES

Why do I need to increase calories during cancer treatment?

Most people with cancer lose weight because they do not eat as much as their bodies need during this time to rebuild healthy tissue injured by surgery, radiation, or chemotherapy. When you eat less, your body uses its own stored fat, protein, and other nutrients for energy. Doctors have found that patients with cancer who maintain their weight and eat diets high in protein and calories during their treatment can better tolerate the side effects of their therapy.

These tips may help if you have appetite loss or weight loss.

- Go nuts! A small handful of nuts contains about 200 calories—a lot of nutrition packed in a small amount of food.
- Make all fluids count! Drink only liquids that contain calories, such as 100% fruit juice, milk, and liquid nutritional supplements. Avoid calorie-free beverages like coffee, tea, and diet soft drinks.
- Sink your teeth into some calories. During mealtime, stick with foods and dishes that contain high amounts of calories. For example, it is okay to eat the main dish plus some fruit, bread, potatoes, and rice. Skip the salad and broth-based soups. These foods normally are very good for you and an important part of a healthy diet. However, if you are having trouble eating enough, these foods will fill you up without providing much-needed calories and protein, so they should be avoided.
- Anything goes! Unless your doctor, nurse, or dietitian has told you to avoid specific foods as part of your treatment, no foods are off limits! This is one time where eating "what is good for you" is not the most important goal. Once you get through treatment and are feeling better, you can shift your focus to healthful eating for the long term.
- Sauce it up! Add sauces or gravies to foods that you eat. These can add a few extra calories to every meal and may make the food more appealing to you. Mash vegetables with milk and add some grated cheese and egg.
- Break tradition! Eat your favorite foods any time of the day. For example, if you like breakfast foods, eat them for dinner or for a snack. Having waffles at

three o'clock in the afternoon is fine if that's what you want!

- Treat food like medication. Set some times to eat, such as every one-half to one hour. Then be sure to have at least one or two bites of food at each "medication" time. Every calorie you eat counts, even if they are spread throughout the day.

- Be a sour puss! If sweet things don't taste good to you, try making a sour, tart, or mildly sweet shake or smoothie. For example, you can make a fruit smoothie or milkshake with frozen cranberries. Or try adding one or two teaspoons of finely ground decaffeinated coffee to a chocolate or vanilla liquid supplement, such as Boost® or Ensure®.

FOOD FOR THOUGHT:

"I use cream cheese and sour cream when I make mashed potatoes for my husband. It adds extra calories, and he likes the creamier potatoes!"

—Ruby J., wife and caregiver

"I put bananas in the freezer and add them to liquid nutritional supplements with ice cream and chocolate syrup. They are delicious and make a thick and creamy shake."

—Pam W., multiple myeloma survivor

ADDING MORE PROTEIN

What foods are high in protein?

Foods that are high in protein include
- Meats—beef, chicken, fish, turkey, pork, and lamb
- Dairy products—cheese, yogurt, cottage cheese, and cream cheese
- Eggs
- Peanut butter and nuts
- Dried beans and peas—kidney beans, black beans, lentils, and chickpeas or hummus

- Soy foods—tofu and soy-based beef, chicken, or sausage substitutes

What are some ways that I can make my favorite foods higher in protein?

- Fortify it! Add nonfat powdered milk, whey protein powder, or soy protein powder to mashed potatoes, macaroni and cheese, casseroles, smoothies, and other soft foods.
- Blend it! Blend a fruit smoothie of bananas, frozen berries, milk, and 1–2 tablespoons of nonfat powdered milk or whey protein powder.
- Substitute it! Use milk instead of water to make hot cereals such as oatmeal or cream of wheat.
- Say cheese! Try cheese (100 calories and 7 grams of protein per ounce) as a snack and in sandwiches. Add it to casseroles, potatoes, and soups, as well!
- Power up your milk! Add one cup of dry milk powder to one quart of whole milk and shake until powder is dissolved (207 calories and 14 grams of protein per serving). Refrigerate and use as you would regular milk.

FOOD FOR THOUGHT:

"I love going to fast-food restaurants and getting a really big milkshake. Not only does it give me extra calories, but it is loaded with extra protein, too. Sometimes I even mix in a protein powder to give it even more protein."

—Joan L., esophageal cancer survivor

"When I make eggs, I always add some shredded cheese to increase the protein content."

—Mary G., lung cancer survivor

- Dip it! Use peanut butter (4 grams of protein per tablespoon), hummus, cream cheese, or cheese spreads on toast, bagels, pretzels, crackers, bananas, apples, and celery. Make nachos with baked tortilla chips, whole beans or fat-free refried beans, cheese, olives, guacamole, and salsa.

RECIPES FOR ADDING MORE CALORIES

WARM BREAKFAST SMOOTHIE

Nothing says "good morning" like a nice warm drink! This one is loaded with fiber, protein, and antioxidants.

Ingredients

½ cup cooked oatmeal (instant, quick, or regular)
½ cup low-fat vanilla yogurt
½ cup brewed green tea

½ cup frozen blueberries, thawed (or other berry)
1–2 oz vanilla protein powder (about 1 scoop) (optional)

Directions

- In a small pot, combine all ingredients. Heat through to desired temperature while mashing berries with the back of a spoon. Serve and enjoy!

Makes 1–2 servings

Nutrition Facts

Per serving: 295 calories, 3 g fat, 26 g protein, 50 g carbohydrates, 6 g fiber, 100 mg sodium

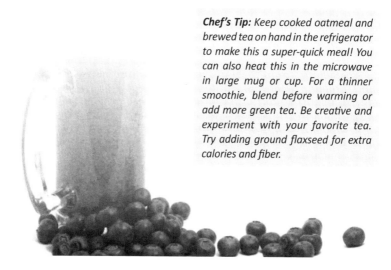

Chef's Tip: *Keep cooked oatmeal and brewed tea on hand in the refrigerator to make this a super-quick meal! You can also heat this in the microwave in large mug or cup. For a thinner smoothie, blend before warming or add more green tea. Be creative and experiment with your favorite tea. Try adding ground flaxseed for extra calories and fiber.*

BLUEBERRY POWER MUFFINS

Big or small, these muffins pack a powerful punch! Fill each muffin tin to the top for bigger muffins; this gives about 14 muffins/batch of batter. Or, you can make mini muffins and snack on several throughout the day.

Ingredients

Dry

2½ cups whole wheat flour
1 cup old-fashioned oats (not the quick kind)
½ cup soya granules
1 scoop vanilla or plain whey protein powder

1 cup sugar
1 tablespoon baking powder
1 teaspoon baking soda
½ teaspoon salt
1 cup chopped almonds

Wet

¾ cup whole milk
½ cup buttermilk
⅓ cup ricotta cheese
2 tablespoons vegetable oil

1 tablespoon vanilla
1 teaspoon almond extract
2 eggs
1⅓ cups blueberries

Directions
- Preheat oven to 400°F.
- Mix dry ingredients in a large bowl.
- Mix wet ingredients, excluding blueberries, in a medium bowl.
- Add wet ingredients to dry ingredients and stir just until mixed.
- Gently stir in blueberries.
- Spoon batter into a muffin pan sprayed with cooking spray. Fill almost to top.
- Bake at 400° for 18–22 minutes. Remove immediately and cool on wire rack.

Makes 20 muffins

Nutrition Facts
Per muffin: 225 calories, 8 g fat, 10 g protein, 30 g carbohydrates, 4 g fiber, 200 mg sodium

RECIPES FOR ADDING MORE PROTEIN

EASY HIGH-PROTEIN SMOOTHIES

These smoothies are like milkshakes, thin or thick, depending on the temperature.

Ingredients

1 cup yogurt   1 cup cottage cheese

Directions
- Add one of the following and blend until smooth:
  - 1 banana + several strawberries + 1 teaspoon vanilla + honey to taste or
  - 1 peach + several strawberries + 1 teaspoon vanilla + honey to taste or
  - 1 banana + 2 tablespoons peanut butter + 1 teaspoon vanilla + honey to taste
- Variations: Add your favorite fruit or jam. Substitute chocolate or other flavoring for vanilla. For a thinner texture, add milk or more yogurt. If you prefer it colder, blend with ice cubes.

Makes 1 serving

Nutrition Facts
Per serving: 600 calories, 24 g fat, 43 g protein, 79 g carbohydrates, 5 g fiber, 1,000 mg sodium

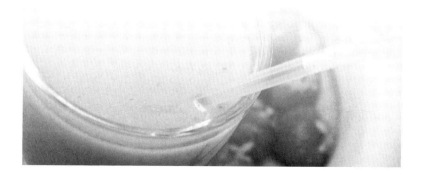

WHOLE WHEAT MACARONI AND CHEESE BAKE

This mac and cheese requires a little more work but is well worth it. The hidden vegetables in the dish are a healthy and tasty surprise. You can use more whole milk instead of broth for higher calories.

Ingredients

1 cup white or yellow onion, chopped

1 cup vegetable mix: chopped celery, cooked carrot, orange bell pepper, butternut squash

1 cup cauliflower, chopped

2 tablespoons olive oil

2 tablespoons flour

½ teaspoon salt

¼ teaspoon garlic

¼ teaspoon white pepper

¼ teaspoon paprika

1 cup chicken or vegetable broth

1 cup whole milk

2 cups cheddar cheese, shredded

5 cups cooked whole wheat macaroni pasta (2½ cups uncooked)

⅓ cup coarse bread crumbs, any type

½ teaspoon dried thyme (optional)

Directions

- Preheat oven to 425°F.
- Heat olive oil in a nonstick skillet over medium heat. Add vegetables and cook until tender. Stir in flour and cook about 1–2 minutes.
- Slowly add stock and milk to skillet, stirring to prevent lumps. Add spices and cook until heated through.
- Puree mixture in blender or food processor. Return mixture to pot, add cheese, and heat until melted thoroughly. Add cooked macaroni and stir to combine.
- Spread macaroni in a medium baking dish coated with nonstick spray. Top with bread crumbs and thyme.
- Bake for 10 minutes or until topping is golden.
- Allow to rest for a few minutes before serving, and enjoy with your favorite vegetable side.

Makes 6 servings

Nutrition Facts

Per serving: 450 calories, 22 g fat, 19 g protein, 26 g carbohydrates, 5 g fiber, 338 mg sodium

PEANUT BUTTER OATMEAL COOKIES

These cookies are tasty, wholesome treats. They are a good source of protein, essential fatty acids, and whole grains. They make a fun breakfast or quick snack.

Ingredients

1 cup natural peanut butter
1 cup brown sugar
½ cup low-fat vanilla yogurt
2 eggs
2 teaspoons vanilla extract
2 cups oats
⅓ cup flaxseed meal
1½ cups white whole wheat flour or all-purpose flour

½ cup vanilla soy protein
1 teaspoon baking powder
½ teaspoon baking soda
1 teaspoon salt
½ cup dark chocolate chips (optional)

Directions

- Preheat oven to 350°F. Spray cookie sheet with nonstick cooking spray.
- In a large bowl, beat together peanut butter, brown sugar, yogurt, eggs, and vanilla until light and fluffy.
- In a medium bowl, combine oats, flaxseed, flour, protein powder, baking powder, baking soda, salt, and chocolate chips, if using.
- Stir dry ingredients into peanut butter mixture until well combined.
- Place rounded tablespoons of cookie dough onto prepared cookie sheet. Flatten cookies with fork, and bake for 12–15 minutes.
- Remove to cooling rack. Cookies will be chewy in center.

Makes 30 servings

Nutrition Facts

Per serving (1 cookie): 181 calories, 7 g fat, 7 g protein, 24 g carbohydrates, 3 g fiber, 114 mg sodium

CHAPTER 6

FIGHTING INFECTIONS

P eople with cancer are at a higher risk of developing infections because they tend to have weakened immune systems. You can do a few things to help lessen the chance of getting an infection. Some foods may cause illness if not properly prepared. To avoid getting a food-borne illness, it is best to always follow food safety guidelines.

LOW WHITE BLOOD CELL COUNTS

What is neutropenia?

Neutropenia is a condition in which the number of neutrophils, a type of white blood cell, is abnormally low. Neutropenia can be a side effect of some types of cancer treatments.

What can happen if there is a change in my neutrophil count?

A sudden increase or decrease in your neutrophil count indicates a possible infection. You are at increased risk of developing an infection if your neutrophil level falls below 1,000/mm^3.

What can cause neutropenia?

- Radiation therapy
- Chemotherapy
- Leukemia
- Lymphoma
- Bone marrow transplantation
- Aplastic anemia
- Myelodysplastic syndromes
- Chronic liver disease

What can I do to help prevent the development of infection?

General health:

- Wash your hands frequently with soap and water.
- Avoid contact with people who are a source of infection (such as those with the flu, colds, cold sores, or chicken pox).
- Avoid people who have been recently vaccinated (immunized with a live virus). Speak with your doctor or nurse regarding types of vaccines made from live viruses.
- Keep your mouth, teeth, and gums clean. Use a soft toothbrush and mild saltwater rinses.
- Inspect your mouth daily for sores on the tongue, cheeks, and gums.
- Avoid contact with animals, especially birds and cats, that can transmit viruses. Speak with your healthcare provider about pet care.
- Inspect skin daily for open wounds or cuts.
- Use caution when using sharp objects near the skin, such as kitchen knives and manicure sets.
- Get plenty of sleep each night.

Nutrition-related:

- Include high-protein foods in your diet, such as properly cooked eggs, chicken, fish, beans, and tofu.
- Eat high-calorie foods to maintain energy levels and prevent weight loss, such as whole milk, cheese, milkshakes, meats, and peanut butter.
- Include foods with vitamin C, such as fruits and fruit juice and vegetables.
- Drink plenty of fluids.

Basic food safety guidelines to help prevent food-borne illness:
- Always wash hands before and after handling or preparing food.
- Keep work areas, cutting boards, and cutting utensils clean and sanitized. Use separate cutting boards for raw meats and cooked foods.
- Do not buy foods in damaged or dented containers.
- Keep perishable foods cold (40°F and below) and keep hot foods hot (140°F and above).
- Cook all meats well (at least 160°F); use a meat thermometer to make sure.
- Never leave food at room temperature longer than two hours.
- Observe expiration dates on food packages, and discard any foods kept past their expiration date.

What can I do to reduce my risk of infection before surgery?

Major surgery places certain significant nutrient demands on the body as well as exposes the body to serious complications. The use of oral nutrition products containing specific nutrients such as arginine, fish oil, antioxidants, and nucleotides, like Nestlé IMPACT Advance Recovery® formula, have been shown to reduce the risk of hospital-acquired infections and pneumonia, reduce mound complications, and shorten hospital stays in patients undergoing major surgery. Products like these may be useful if you are scheduled for major gastrointestinal or other surgery, as they provide the nutrients needed to support the immune system before and after surgery. Research continues in regard to their routine use, so discuss with your healthcare team to see if they would be right for you (Marik & Zaloga, 2010; Waitzberg, Saito, Plank, Jamieson, & Jagannath, 2006).

What are the basic guidelines for a neutropenic or low-bacteria diet?

- Avoid all uncooked vegetables and most raw fruits. Cooked vegetables, canned fruits, and juices are fine. Choose raw fruits that are thick-skinned and that can be peeled, such as bananas, oranges, and melons. Make sure these fruits are washed in cold water and handled safely. Avoid thin-skinned raw fruits like grapes, plums, and strawberries.
- Avoid raw or rare-cooked meat, fish, and eggs.
- Avoid salad bars, fruit bars, buffets, and deli counters. Buy vacuum-packed lunch meats rather than freshly sliced deli meats.
- Avoid cold soups, such as gazpacho or vichyssoise.
- Avoid soft, mold-ripened and veined cheeses, including Brie, Camembert, Roquefort, Stilton, Gorgonzola, and blue.
- You may drink tap water or bottled water. Well water can be used if boiled for one minute before using.

PREVENTING FOOD-BORNE ILLNESS

Cancer therapy can weaken the immune system. This means that you can easily "catch a bug" or get an infection. Food is rarely, if ever, the proven source of infection. There appears to be no need to strictly avoid specific foods. It is important, however, to not consume contaminated foods and to follow safe food-handling practices. Avoid eating foods whose preparation and handling are unknown, such as deli sandwiches and fast food.

Fruit and vegetable tips

- Wash fruits and vegetables thoroughly. Use a vegetable brush designed for this purpose.
- Throw out fruits or vegetables with rotten or moldy spots on them.
- Remove peels and outer leaves where possible.

Meat and meat product tips

- Eat fully cooked meats, poultry, fish, and eggs at home and in restaurants.
- Cook red meat, including ground beef, to an internal temperature of at least 160°F.
- Cook fish to 145°F and until the flesh is opaque and flakes with a fork.
- Avoid eating sushi, sashimi, and dishes that contain raw eggs or fish.
- Thaw meat and poultry in the refrigerator, not at room temperature.
- Don't use cracked eggs because they could contain harmful bacteria, viruses, and parasites.
- Avoid stuffing poultry before cooking; instead, cook stuffing separately to ensure safety.

Milk and milk product tips

- Consume only pasteurized milk and cheeses.
- Refrigerate fresh milk and milk products as soon as possible after purchase. Keep poured and unused milk separate; do not pour milk back into original container.
- Once reconstituted, dry milk should be refrigerated.

General tips

- Place raw meats on the bottom shelf of the refrigerator or below cooked or ready-to-eat foods like fruits and lunch meat.
- Maintain foods at proper temperature. Keep foods out of the danger zone, which is 40°F–140°F. Reheat food to at least 165°F to lower bacterial growth.
- Microwave foods thoroughly according to directions, in a covered dish, and observing standing times.
- When shopping, make sure frozen foods are solid and refrigerated foods are cold.
- Make frozen and refrigerated foods the last purchase on your shopping list, especially during the summer months.
- Date leftovers so that you make sure to use them within a day or two.
- Never use food from cans that are cracked, bulging, or leaking or that spurt liquid when opened.
- Use clean towels and dish cloths. Change them often or use disposable paper towels.
- Adhere to good personal hygiene, such as
  - Wash hands before preparing or handling food, after using the toilet, and after touching any soiled object.
  - Wear clean aprons and clean outer garments during food handling.

REFERENCES

Marik, P.E., & Zaloga, G.P. (2010). Immunonutrition in high-risk surgical patients: A systematic review and analysis of the literature. *Journal of Parenteral and Enteral Nutrition, 34,* 378–386. doi:10.1177/0148607110362692

Waitzberg, D.L., Saito, H., Plank, L.D., Jamieson, G.G., & Jagannath, P. (2006). Postsurgical infections are reduced with specialized nutrition support. *World Journal of Surgery, 30,* 1592–1604.

RECIPES

CHICKEN SALAD WITH CRANBERRIES AND WALNUTS

A quick and easy lunch that requires minimal work. It's tasty and high in protein. Great in a sandwich, with crackers, or on your favorite salad greens.

Ingredients

1 10-oz can chicken chunks, drained

½ cup diced celery

2 tablespoons chopped parsley, chives, or your favorite herb

¼ cup nondairy mayonnaise

¼ cup dried cranberries

¼ cup chopped walnuts

Salt and pepper to taste

Directions

- Combine all ingredients in a small bowl.
- Refrigerate until ready to serve.

Makes 4 servings

Nutrition Facts

Per serving: 173 calories, 10.5 g fat, 11 g protein, 9 g carbohydrates, 0.5 g fiber, 280 mg sodium

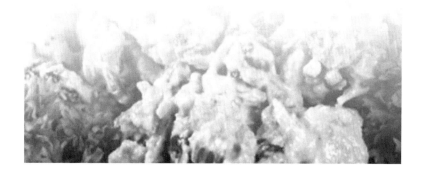

SIMPLE WHITE CHICKEN CHILI

A savory and flavorful, yet light, chili. It makes a great meal for stocking the freezer. Just divide chili among individual containers, date, and label; they will be a quick and easy meal. Thaw overnight in the refrigerator or defrost in the microwave.

Ingredients

- 1 medium onion, diced
- 1 green bell pepper, diced
- 2 tablespoons olive oil
- 1 tablespoon minced garlic (or ½ teaspoon garlic powder, added with other spices)
- 1 teaspoon dried thyme
- 1 teaspoon cumin
- 1 teaspoon white or black pepper
- 1 teaspoon salt (optional)
- 2 14-oz cans of white beans, drained, or 1 cup dry beans, soaked and cooked
- 2 cups chicken broth or water
- 1 10-oz can chicken chunks, drained
- Pinch of cayenne pepper or hot sauce to taste

Directions

- Sauté vegetables and garlic (if using fresh) in a medium pot with olive oil on medium heat until vegetables and garlic become soft, about 5–8 minutes.
- Add seasonings to the sautéed vegetables and garlic; mix well.
- Add cooked beans, chicken, and broth to the pot and let it simmer for 15 minutes with the lid on.

Makes 6 servings

Nutrition Facts

Per serving: 170 calories, 7 g fat, 14 g protein, 20 g carbohydrates, 6.5 g fiber, 62 mg sodium

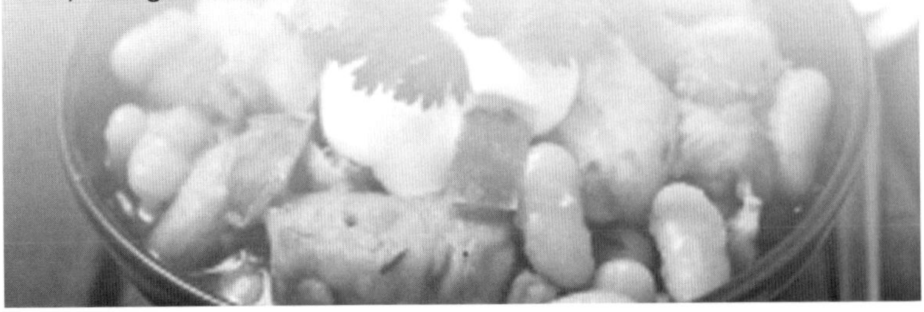

WHOLE WHEAT PITA PIZZAS

Pizza is always a fun meal, especially when you aren't feeling good. These pita pizzas are quick, healthy, and tasty. You can top them with virtually any cheese, meat, and/or vegetable. Experiment with your favorite ingredients! They also keep well in the refrigerator and can be made ahead of time.

Ingredients
- 4 6-inch whole wheat pitas
- 1 cup of your favorite pizza or pasta sauce
- 1½ cups shredded mozzarella cheese
- 1 cup chopped peppers or mushrooms (or a mixture of both)
- ½ cup pepperoni slices, cooked chicken, or cooked sausage

Directions
- Preheat oven to 400°F.
- Spray a baking sheet with cooking spray, and place pitas on sheet.
- Top each pita evenly with sauce, shredded cheese, vegetables, and meat.
- Bake pizza for about 10 minutes or until cheese is browned and bubbly.

Makes 4 servings

Nutrition Facts
Per serving: 449 calories, 19 g fat, 26 g protein, 43 g carbohydrates, 2.5 g fiber, 900 mg sodium

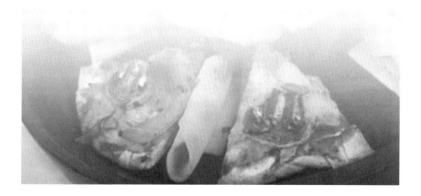

RED "REFRIED" BEANS

Beans, or any legume, are high in protein, fiber, and essential nutrients. These "from-scratch" beans require little attention and are an inexpensive addition to any meal. Serve along eggs or rice, or top with shredded cheese and salsa. They are flavorful and will surely awaken your taste buds.

Ingredients

1 cup red beans, dried (sort through beans to remove any pebbles or distorted beans)
½ onion, cut in a large dice
1 teaspoon kosher salt
1 bay leaf, small
1 teaspoon cumin
1 teaspoon fine-ground black pepper

1 teaspoon chipotle peppers, minced
2 tablespoons olive oil
½ teaspoon paprika
½ teaspoon garlic, granulated
¼ teaspoon salt (optional)
2 tablespoons tomato puree

Directions

- In a medium heat-proof bowl, soak beans in about 4 cups of hot water for 10 minutes.
- Drain and repeat, conserving the soaking liquid.
- In a medium pot, add beans, soaking liquid, onions, bay leaf, and salt.
- Simmer on low for 1½–2 hours or until beans are tender.
- Cool slightly and drain. Add spices, chipotles, oil, and tomato.
- Puree in food processor, or mash with potato masher.

Makes 4 servings

Nutrition Facts
Per serving: 204 calories, 8 g fat, 12 g protein, 31 g carbohydrates, 12 g fiber, 311 mg sodium

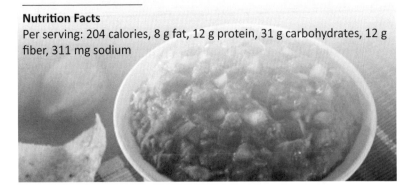

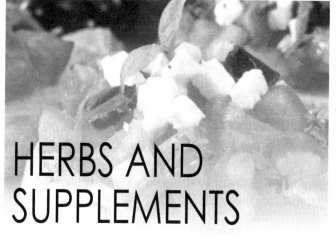

CHAPTER 7

HERBS AND SUPPLEMENTS

M illions of people use a variety of herbs and supplements in their quest for health, including a significant percentage of people with cancer. Today's dietary supplements are found in many different forms, and although there is scientific evidence supporting the benefits of some dietary supplements, such as specific vitamins or minerals for certain health conditions, the use of dietary supplements in cancer care needs further research.

It is important to know that herbal and vitamin supplements do not have to be approved by the U.S. Food and Drug Administration (FDA) in order to be marketed and sold to consumers. Manufacturers are free to make statements and testimonial claims about these products without a full course of research and clinical trials. The labels of nutritional supplements like herbs and vitamins will clearly state that the product is not intended to diagnose, treat, cure, or prevent any disease and that any statements made have not been evaluated by the FDA. Herbal and vitamin supplements are not held to the same standards as drugs and are thus not routinely monitored. Supplement manufacturers routinely, and legally, can sell their products without first having to demonstrate that they are safe and effective.

Many people assume that herbs and supplements are "natural" and therefore "safe," but there are many situations—particularly for patients receiving chemotherapy—where this assumption can be dangerous. Following are some of the known problems associated with herbs and supplements when combined with cancer treatments.

- Studies have shown that some herbs, especially St. John's wort, may interfere with the effectiveness of some chemotherapy medicines used to treat cancer. Dietary supplements have the potential to make medications more effective or less effective. Neither is good. Making chemotherapy more effective may increase the toxic side effects that are often experienced with treatments, and certainly, no one wants the treatments to be less effective.

- Although there are benefits to eating foods high in antioxidants, the use of high doses of antioxidant vitamins like vitamins A, C, and E has not shown increased protection from cancer. In fact, studies have shown that beta-carotene supplements can actually increase the risk of lung and prostate cancer in smokers. These vitamins may also have a protective effect on all cells, including cancer cells, thus making treatments less effective.

- Many herbal products and soy supplements have an estrogen-like effect on the body and should be avoided by women with estrogen receptor–positive breast cancer.

- Other herbs, such as dong quai, feverfew, ginkgo, ginseng, and St. John's wort, may lower blood platelet levels, causing excessive bleeding if taken in high doses.

- Remember that just because an herb is classified as "natural" does not mean that it is either helpful or healthy.
- Of the top best-selling dietary supplements in the United States, nine have been determined to pose a possible risk when taken with specific chemotherapy medications or specific cancer treatments. These include
  – Echinacea
  – Garlic
  – Ginkgo
  – Ginseng
  – Grapeseed
  – Kava
  – Soy supplements
  – St. John's wort
  – Valerian.

What is a phytochemical?
Phytochemicals refer to the wide variety of "good" chemicals found in plants. They are generally found in fruits, vegetables, beans, grains, and other plants. Thousands of phytochemicals have been identified in foods that have either antioxidant or hormone-like actions. Phytochemicals and antioxidants are often associated with cancer protection because of their ability to protect the cells in our bodies from the damage of free radicals.

The preferred choice to meet all of your nutritional needs is from food that you consume on a daily basis. Eating a variety of fruits, vegetables, and whole grains will provide all of the vitamins, minerals, and phytochemicals needed to help your body fight cancer. Research continues to determine the safety and possible benefits of using herbs, antioxidants, vitamins, and minerals during cancer treatment. The jury is still out, but most medical experts agree that you should avoid high doses of nutritional supplements or herbs, as not enough is known about their potential impact on cancer therapies. Most of the more positive results showing the benefits of herb and supplement use have been seen in animal studies and not human studies. There just is not enough consistent and significant data at this time to recommend the use of supplements in cancer care.

Talk to your healthcare team if you are taking or are considering taking herbs or supplements, especially while you are undergoing treatment for cancer. Although research shows that most patients do not feel comfortable discussing these issues with their physicians, healthcare professionals are becoming more knowledgeable and supportive in helping their patients make informed choices in regard to complementary and alternative therapies.

Eating healthfully during treatment is important to the healing process. Your body needs a wide variety of nutrients to feel good and recover. Although it is safe to eat nutrient-rich foods, such as vegetables and fruit, it may not be safe to take the nutrients themselves as dietary supplements.

What is açai berry?

This fruit has been growing in popularity over the past few years. Açai (pronounced ah-sah-EE) berry is the fruit of the açai palm, native to Central and South America. The berry's popularity has led to this fruit being manufactured in many forms such as juices and freeze-dried açai supplements with health claims ranging from weight loss to cancer prevention. The benefit of açai berry appears to come from its high antioxidant level. Studies confirm that the fruit does exhibit some antioxidant activity, but the conclusions found regarding the specific potency vary from study to study. In fact, some studies demonstrated that açai berry juice had less antioxidant activity than red wine, strawberries, grapes, and pomegranate juice.

The bottom line is that, like most other fruits, açai berry contains antioxidants, but there is no clear evidence that this exotic fruit is more healthful than any other. Whole fruits, rather than their juice, will provide you with more fiber and often less calories. And there is no clear health benefit to recommend freeze-dried fruit supplement pills.

RECIPES

VEGETABLE SOUP

Fruits and vegetables seem to play an important part in lowering the incidence of many cancers. Because they contain important phytochemicals and antioxidants that protect our cells from damage, it is very important to eat a variety of fruits and vegetables—more than five a day . . . every day!

Ingredients

- ⅔ cup sliced carrots
- ½ cup diced onions
- 1½ cup diced cabbage
- ½ cup green beans
- 2 cloves garlic, minced
- 3 cups chicken, beef, or vegetable broth

- 1 tablespoon tomato paste
- ½ teaspoon basil
- ¼ teaspoon oregano
- ½ cup diced zucchini

Directions

- In a large saucepan sprayed with nonstick cooking spray, sauté carrots, onion, and garlic over low heat until tender, about 5 minutes.
- Add broth, cabbage, beans, tomato paste, and spices, and bring to a boil.
- Lower heat and simmer, covered, 15–20 minutes or until the beans are tender.
- Stir in zucchini and heat 3–4 minutes longer.

Makes 4 servings

Nutrition Facts
Per serving: 60 calories, 1 g fat, 5 g protein, 8 g carbohydrates, 2 g fiber, 595 mg sodium

TOMATO BRUSCHETTA

Live it up with lycopene, an antioxidant found in tomatoes and tomato-based foods. High intake of tomato-based foods has been shown to reduce the risk of some cancers, especially those of the prostate. Lycopene is activated in the cooking process, so raw, fresh tomatoes will not provide the lycopene your body needs.

Ingredients

1 loaf of French or Italian bread

2 tablespoons softened margarine

1 cup diced tomatoes, fresh or canned

¼ cup sliced ripe olives

½ teaspoon basil leaves

¾ cup crumbled feta cheese

2 cloves garlic, chopped

¼ cup canola or olive oil

Directions

- Preheat oven to 375°F. Cut bread loaf horizontally in half. Place halves, cut sides up, on a cookie sheet.
- Brush bread with softened margarine, and top with tomatoes, olives, basil, and feta cheese.
- Mix garlic and oil, and drizzle over the cheese.
- Bake 15 minutes or until cheese just begins to brown.
- Cut into slices and enjoy!

Makes 20 servings

Nutrition Facts

Per serving (1 slice): 75 calories, 5 g fat, 2 g protein, 5 g carbohydrates, 0 g fiber, 153 mg sodium

MANDARIN ORANGE SALAD

Vitamin C is found in many fruits and vegetables, especially citrus fruits. Many studies have linked a high intake of vitamin C–rich foods with a reduced risk of cancer.

Ingredients

Salad

- 1 head Romaine lettuce, torn into pieces
- 1 cup celery, chopped
- ¼ cup slivered almonds
- 2 tablespoons green onion, thinly sliced
- 1 can (11 oz) mandarin orange segments

Dressing

- ¼ cup canola oil
- 2 tablespoons vinegar
- 1 tablespoon sugar
- Salt and pepper to taste

Directions

- Mix salad greens, celery, slivered almonds, and onion together.
- Combine all salad dressing ingredients, and shake or stir until mixed well.
- Add dressing to salad, and mix until well coated.
- Right before serving, add drained mandarin orange segments.

Makes 6 servings

Nutrition Facts

Per serving (1 cup): 140 calories, 11 g fat, 2 g protein, 10 g carbohydrates, 2 g fiber, 25 mg sodium

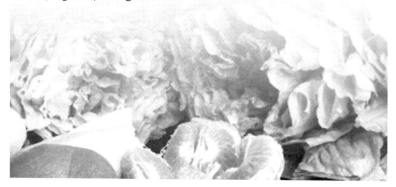

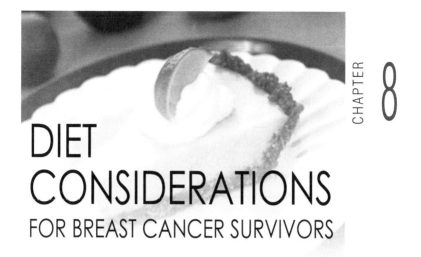

CHAPTER 8

DIET CONSIDERATIONS
FOR BREAST CANCER SURVIVORS

U nlike many cancers, in which weight loss can be a significant side effect, women with breast cancer can sometimes gain weight during cancer treatment. This may be caused by hormonal changes, medications, changes in activity, emotional changes, or a combination of these factors. Following the tips in this chapter may help prevent you from gaining unwanted weight and help keep you healthy for years to come!

EAT MORE FRUITS AND VEGETABLES

- Fruits and vegetables are excellent sources of fiber, vitamins, minerals, and phytochemicals. These "good plant chemicals," found naturally in all fruits and vegetables, may offer better protection against cancer cells than what would be received by taking a vitamin supplement alone.
- Fruits and vegetables are generally lower in calories than foods from other food groups and make great snacks to satisfy hunger, if needed.

- Variety is the key, and the more colorful, the better! Choose dark-orange, green, red, and purple fruits and vegetables such as sweet potatoes, spinach, beets, red peppers, strawberries, raspberries, and blueberries.

CHOOSE THE RIGHT FATS

- Did you know there are good fats and bad fats? Fats that come from animal sources are thought to be more harmful than fats from vegetable sources, such as avocados and olives. A plant-based diet that limits animal fats is part of a healthy cancer prevention diet.
- Some research suggests that fish oil, especially omega-3 fatty acids, may reduce the risk of breast cancer by helping to improve the immune system. Some foods high in omega-3 fatty acids include seafoods such as shellfish, tuna, salmon, mackerel, trout, and sardines. Other foods high in omega-3s include canola oil, flaxseed, wheat germ, almonds, and soybeans.
- Remember that regardless of the source, fat adds calories to the diet, and too many calories will lead to unwanted weight gain.

FILL UP ON FIBER

- Dietary fiber is the part of the food, usually from plant sources, that is not digested.
- A diet rich in fiber promotes a feeling of fullness, making it easier to maintain your weight because you may eat less.
- Aim for 25–35 grams of fiber daily from whole grain breads and cereals, dried beans, nuts, and fresh fruits and vegetables.

WATCH THE SUGAR

- Many cancer survivors will hear that sugar "feeds" cancer and it must be avoided. The bottom line is that sugar feeds *every* cell in the body to provide a source of energy. Avoiding all sugar, however, will not prevent the cancer from growing. Sugar is a form of carbohydrate, and carbohydrates are also found in many healthy foods, such as fruits, vegetables, and whole grains.

- Consuming simple sugars in the form of desserts, candy, and soft drinks not only increases the calories in your diet but also provides no nourishment for your healthy cells. By eating "good" complex carbohydrates such as whole grains, fruits, and vegetables, you can actually increase the amount of the cancer-fighting phytochemicals in your diet, which is beneficial, not harmful.

- Eating simple sugars may also increase levels of certain hormones, like insulin, in the body. It is these hormones, not the actual sugar, that appear to fuel cancer cell growth. So, by achieving an ideal weight for your body type and avoiding high-fat, high-sugar foods, you may be able to decrease the insulin hormone level in your body and reduce cancer cell growth.

BONE UP ON CALCIUM

- Bone loss can be a long-term effect of chemotherapy as well as an effect of the reduced estrogen production that is often seen in postmenopausal women.

- Many patients with breast cancer are not permitted to take estrogen replacement medications, so it is important to receive enough calcium through the diet to prevent osteoporosis.

- It is best to prevent bone loss before it occurs rather than to treat osteoporosis later in life. Adequate calcium intake, from diet or supplements, as well as adequate exercise will enhance and maintain bone density.
- Recommended intake of calcium is 1,500 mg each day.

Food Sources of Calcium

High (250–350 mg calcium)	Moderate (100–200 mg calcium)	Low (50–100 mg calcium)
• 1 cup milk	• ½ cup turnip greens	• ½ cup broccoli
• 1 cup yogurt	• 1 cup cottage cheese	• ½ cup ice cream
• 1 cup calcium-fortified juice	• 3 oz tofu	• ½ cup pinto beans, chickpeas, or navy beans
• 1 cup calcium-fortified soy or rice milk	• ½ cup white beans	• ½ cup kale, okra, or bok choy
• 1 oz cheese	• 3 oz canned salmon	• 2 dried figs
• 3 oz canned sardines	• ¼ cup almonds	• 1 cup whole wheat flour
		• 1 tablespoon molasses

BE SENSIBLE WITH SOY

- Laboratory studies looking at soy's effect on breast cancer cells have shown mixed results. The active chemicals that are naturally found in soy are called *isoflavones*. In laboratory studies, these isoflavones act like estrogens, sometimes accelerating the growth of cancer cells. Human studies, however, have not shown the same results. Because of conflicting studies, experts are uncertain if soy has a positive or negative effect on breast cancer cells.

- Most experts report that eating small amounts (3–5 servings per week) of soy foods is safe for breast cancer survivors. Foods containing soy, such as tofu, soybeans, textured vegetable protein, soy milk, and soy nuts, can be part of a healthy cancer prevention diet.
- If you have been diagnosed with an estrogen receptor–positive cancer, do not use soy supplements in the form of pills or powders. The isoflavone concentration is too high, and this may have an unwanted estrogen effect on the body.
- If you take estrogen-blocking medications such as tamoxifen, you should limit your intake of soy foods and avoid soy supplements. Because soy can act in the same way as estrogen, there is a worry that increasing soy in the diet may decrease the effectiveness of these drugs.
- Research is inconclusive, and studies are ongoing. Until more research is available, it is best to be cautious in your use of soy.

HERBAL SUPPLEMENTS

It is the general feeling that if something is natural, such as an herb, it is safe. However, this is not necessarily true. The truth is that some dietary supplements, natural or otherwise, can interact with your cancer medications, making them either less effective or more toxic to you. This may worsen side effects and result in you receiving less than the full benefits of your cancer treatment.

The dietary supplement industry is nearly unregulated, with little quality control in their production.

Most of the "research" that supports supplement use is observational only and includes testimonials from others claiming their value instead of published clinical trials.

Research is ongoing, and as new information is published, new guidelines for their use will become available. It is important to discuss any dietary supplements that you currently use or are planning to use with your entire healthcare team. They can help guide you and provide you with evidence-based research to support their use.

Herbs and Hot Flashes
Black cohosh
- This is one of the most popular herbs used to treat hot flashes. Most studies to date have shown conflicting results, and although some studies have demonstrated significant reduction in symptoms, most of these were not well-controlled, randomized scientific studies. Research is ongoing to determine if the use of this herb is effective against hot flashes and other menopausal symptoms.
- Because of its estrogenic effect, black cohosh is not recommended for use by women who have estrogen-related cancers.
- Its use may interfere with some chemotherapy medications.
- Some potential side effects include mild stomach upset, headaches, vomiting, and dizziness. Use of this herb also has been associated with an increased risk for liver damage.

St. John's wort
- To date, the research using St. John's wort alone for alleviating hot flashes in postmenopausal women with a history of breast cancer has not demonstrated significant benefits.
- The use of St. John's wort by women being treated for cancer has been discouraged.
- Numerous studies have demonstrated that St. John's wort can negatively interact with many medications, including several that are commonly used in cancer treatments, such as tamoxifen.

Red clover

- The majority of studies measuring red clover's effectiveness on hot flashes suggest that it is not helpful for reducing menopause-related hot flashes.
- Because of its estrogenic effect, red clover is not recommended for use by women with estrogen-related cancers.
- Although red clover is generally considered safe to take, it may have blood-thinning effects and is therefore not recommended for those taking medications like warfarin, which also helps to thin the blood.
- Red clover can also interact with some other medications, making them less effective.

Chaste tree berry

- This plant is most often recommended for relieving symptoms related to premenstrual syndromes.
- Small, uncontrolled studies suggest it may be effective for relieving menopausal symptoms, but sufficient, controlled research is still needed to verify its use.
- It is not recommended for use by women with estrogen-related cancers.
- This herb may interact with several medications, including tamoxifen and anastrozole.
- General side effects include nausea, itching, rash, and headaches.

RECIPES

CARIBBEAN SALMON STEAK

Adding more seafood to your diet will not only reduce the total fat content and ultimately the calorie content but also will provide your body with some much-needed omega-3 fatty acids. Research has indicated that this type of "good" fat may reduce the risk for developing heart disease and certain cancers. Food sources include fish, especially salmon, trout, and sardines, as well as some nuts like almonds and walnuts.

Ingredients

1 navel orange	2 tablespoons red wine vinegar
1 small grapefruit	1 tablespoon olive oil
1 tomato, diced	¼ teaspoon garlic powder
¼ cup diced red onion	½ teaspoon parsley
1 small jalapeno, seeded and finely chopped	4 salmon steaks
	Lemon juice

Directions

- Peel and dice orange and grapefruit.
- In a medium bowl, combine all ingredients except salmon and lemon juice, and refrigerate until salmon is ready to serve.
- Preheat grill or broiler. Brush salmon steaks with lemon juice, and grill or broil about 5 minutes on each side or until flaky.
- Spoon chilled fruit salsa over salmon and serve!

Makes 4 servings

Nutrition Facts
Per serving: 300 calories, 17 g fat, 26 g protein, 10 g carbohydrates, 2 g fiber, 70 mg sodium

KEY LIME PIE

Research shows that low-fat, calcium-rich dairy foods can be a part of a healthy diet and help to achieve your weight loss goals. Dietary calcium can help prevent bone loss and osteoporosis in women. This recipe provides a great way to get some added calcium in a low-fat, low-calorie dessert.

Ingredients

- 1 reduced-fat graham cracker crumb crust
- 1 tablespoon lime juice
- 1½ teaspoons unflavored gelatin
- 2 tablespoons water
- 3 containers (8 oz each) lime-flavored low-fat yogurt
- 4 oz fat-free cream cheese, softened
- ½ cup reduced-fat whipped topping
- 2 teaspoons grated lime peel

Directions

- Mix water and lime juice in a small saucepan.
- Add gelatin by sprinkling on top of liquid in pan. Let stand 1 minute, then heat over low heat, stirring constantly until gelatin dissolves. Set aside to cool slightly.
- In a medium bowl, beat cream cheese until smooth. Add yogurt and lime juice mixture, beating until well blended.
- Fold in whipped topping and lime peel.
- Pour into crust and refrigerate until set. Cut into 8 slices and serve.

Makes 8 servings

Nutrition Facts

Per serving: 160 calories, 4 g fat, 5 g protein, 26 g carbohydrates, 0 g fiber, 200 mg sodium

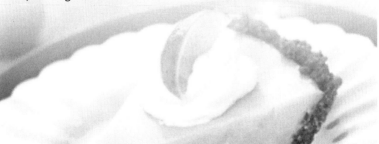

SOUTHWESTERN WRAPS

Obesity has been associated with an increased risk of some cancers. It also appears that the type of fat is more of a concern than the total fat intake. Fat that comes from animal sources may be more of a problem than fat from vegetable oils. Regardless of the source of the fat, it is important to know that fat adds calories and eating too many calories contributes to obesity. This low-fat sandwich is a great alternative to your regular luncheon fare!

Ingredients

3 oz fat-free or light cream cheese

2 tablespoons salsa

2 tablespoons sliced green onion

1 teaspoon Dijon mustard

4 8-inch whole wheat tortillas

1½ cups spinach leaves, washed

8 oz lean sliced turkey breast

¼ cup shredded low-fat cheese

1 medium-sized red bell pepper, sliced

Directions

- Combine cream cheese, salsa, onion, and mustard in a small bowl until well blended and creamy.
- Spread 2 tablespoons mixture over each tortilla.
- Layer spinach, 2 oz turkey, shredded cheese, and red peppers onto each tortilla.
- Roll each tortilla to enclose filling.

Makes 4 servings

Nutrition Facts
Per serving: 214 calories, 5 g fat, 18 g protein, 19 g carbohydrates, 9 g fiber, 930 mg sodium

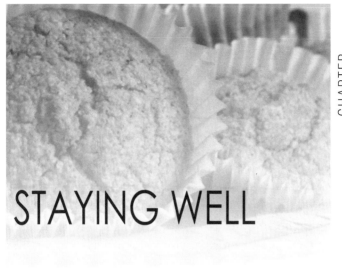

CHAPTER 9

STAYING WELL

Once treatment for your cancer is completed and the symptoms begin to diminish, you can begin to reintroduce some of the foods that you may have eliminated in your diet because of the side effects of your treatments. Cancer survivors may have weakened immune systems for a significant period of time after treatment. A healthy diet with adequate nutrients will help you regain your strength, heal any damaged cells, and help you to feel better each day! Nutrition guidelines for cancer survivors follow the same basic principles proposed for cancer prevention and risk reduction for all Americans. Among those recommendations are the American Cancer Society (ACS) Guidelines on Nutrition and Physical Activity for Cancer Prevention*, which are summarized here.

1. Maintain a healthy weight throughout life.
   - Balance calorie intake with physical activity.
   - Avoid excessive weight gain throughout life.
   - Achieve and maintain a healthy weight if currently overweight or obese.
2. Adopt a physically active lifestyle.

- Engage in at least 30 minutes of moderate to vig-
  orous physical activity, above usual activities, on
  five or more days of the week; 45–60 minutes of
  intentional physical activity is preferable.
3. Eat a healthy diet, with an emphasis on plant
   sources.
   - Choose foods and drinks in amounts that help
     you achieve and maintain a healthy weight.
   - Eat five or more servings of a variety of vegetables
     and fruits every day.
   - Choose whole grains over processed (refined)
     grains.
   - Limit intake of processed and red meats.
4. If you drink alcoholic beverages, limit your intake
   (no more than one drink per day for women or two
   per day for men).

*This summary is a condensed version of the article describing the American
Cancer Society Nutrition and Physical Activity Guidelines, which are updated
every five years. The guidelines were developed by the American Cancer Society 2006 Nutrition and Physical Activity Guidelines Advisory Committee and
approved by the American Cancer Society National Board of Directors on May
19, 2006. The full article, written for healthcare professionals, is published in
the September/October 2006 issue of *CA: A Cancer Journal for Clinicians* and
is available for free online at http://caonline.amcancersoc.org/content/vol56/
issue5/

Frequently Asked Questions

1. Will eating less total fat lower the risk of cancer recurrence or improve survival?

Several studies have looked at the link between fat intake and
survival after the diagnosis of breast cancer, with mixed results.
Although there is little evidence that total fat intake affects cancer
outcomes, diets high in fat tend to be high in calories. High-fat,
high-calorie diets contribute to obesity. Obesity has been linked to
increased cancer risk at several sites, increased risk of recurrence,
and reduced chances of survival for many cancer sites.

2. Can dietary fiber prevent cancer or improve cancer survival?

Dietary fiber includes a wide array of plant carbohydrates that are not digested by the human body. Fibers are either "soluble" (like oat bran) or "insoluble" (like wheat bran and cellulose). Soluble fiber helps lower the risk of heart disease by reducing blood cholesterol levels. Fiber is also linked with improved bowel function. Good sources of fiber are beans, vegetables, whole grains, and fruits.

Links between fiber and cancer risk are weak, but eating fiber-rich foods is still recommended because they contain other nutrients that may help reduce cancer risk and provide other health benefits, such as reduced risk of heart disease. Diets with higher intakes of dietary fiber tend to be lower in overall calories, resulting in healthier weights in people who consume more dietary fiber.

3. Does being overweight increase the risk of cancer recurrence or getting another cancer?

More and more evidence suggests that being overweight raises the risk for recurrence and reduces the odds of survival for many cancers. Increased body weight has been linked with higher death rates for all cancers combined. It has also been linked with increased risk for cancers of the esophagus, colon and rectum, liver, gallbladder, pancreas, and kidney; cancers of the stomach and prostate in men and cancers of the breast, uterus, cervix, and ovary in women; and non-Hodgkin lymphoma and multiple myeloma.

Because of the other proven health benefits to being at a healthy weight, people who are overweight are encouraged to lose weight and maintain a healthy weight. Avoiding weight gain as an adult is important to reduce not only cancer incidence and risk of recurrence but also the risk of other chronic diseases.

4. Are foods labeled "organic" recommended for cancer survivors?

The term *organic* is often used to identify plant foods grown without pesticides and genetic modifications and for meat, poultry, eggs, and dairy products that come from animals that are given no antibiotics or growth hormones. Use of the term *organic* on food labels is regulated by the U.S. Department of Agriculture. The common belief is that organic foods may be more healthful because they reduce an individual's exposure to some chemicals. Organic and nonorganic foods are equal in nutrient content. What makes them different is that organic foods are grown without synthetic fertilizers or chemical pesticides, whereas nonorganic foods may contain small amounts of residues. At this time, no studies in humans exist to show whether such foods are better at reducing cancer risk, recurrence, or progression than foods made by other farming and production methods.

5. Will eating vegetables and fruits lower the risk of cancer recurrence?

Eating more vegetables and fruits has been linked in most studies with a lower risk of lung, oral, esophageal, stomach, and colon cancer. But few studies have been done on whether a diet including many vegetables and fruits can reduce the risk of cancer recurrence or improve survival. Some recent studies have suggested that increasing intake of vegetables may have a helpful effect on recurrence or survival for breast, prostate, and ovarian cancers, but this is not definite.

Still, cancer survivors should be encouraged to get at least five servings of a variety of vegetables and fruits each day because of their other health benefits. Because it is not known which of the compounds in vegetables and fruits are most protective, the best advice is to eat five or more servings of different kinds of colorful vegetables and fruits each day.

6. What are phytochemicals, and do they reduce cancer risk?

The term *phytochemicals* refers to a wide range of compounds made by plants. Some have either antioxidant or hormone-like actions. Studies looking at the effects of phytochemicals on cancer recurrence or progression are very limited. The data that exist are mixed or come from only a few studies. Eating lots of vegetables and fruits seems to reduce the risk of cancer, so researchers are looking for the specific components that might account for this. At this time, there is no evidence that phytochemicals taken as supplements are as helpful as the vegetables, fruits, beans, and grains they come from.

7. Would survivors benefit from taking vitamin and mineral supplements?

During and after cancer treatment, there is a probable benefit of taking a standard multivitamin and mineral supplement that contains about 100% of the daily values because during these times, it may be hard to eat a diet with enough of these nutrients. The use of very large doses of vitamins, minerals, and other dietary supplements is not recommended because evidence exists that some high-dose supplements may actually increase cancer risk.

8. Can nutritional supplements lower cancer risk or the risk of recurrence?

There is strong evidence that a diet rich in vegetables, fruits, and other plant-based foods may reduce the risk of some types of cancer. And some recent studies suggest there may be a helpful effect on recurrence or survival for breast, prostate, and ovarian cancers. But there is no evidence at this time that supplements can provide these benefits. Many healthful compounds are found in vegetables and fruits, and it is likely that these compounds work together to exert their helpful effects. Whole foods are likely to contain important, but as of yet unknown, compounds that are not in supplements. Food is the best source of vitamins and minerals.

RECIPES

ITALIAN PASTA AND BEAN SOUP

Beans and peas, also known as legumes, are a great source of fiber and vegetable protein. They can play an important role as part of a diet to lower cancer risk. Legumes are naturally low in fat and sodium and have no cholesterol! Try adding some of the many varieties of legumes in soups, stews, or casseroles as a replacement for meat.

Ingredients

- ½ cup dried pinto beans
- ½ cup dried kidney beans
- ½ cup dried small white Northern beans
- 1 cup small bowtie pasta
- 2 tablespoons parsley
- 4 chicken-flavored bouillon cubes
- 1 cup chopped onion
- 2 teaspoons dried rosemary
- 1 teaspoon dried basil
- ½ teaspoon minced garlic
- ¼ teaspoon crushed red pepper
- 1 can (28 oz) crushed tomatoes
- 1 cup diced carrots
- 1 cup diced celery

Directions

- Rinse and clean beans. Place in a large pot with 3 cups of water.
- Cover and bring to a boil for 2 minutes.
- Remove from heat and let soak for 1 hour. Drain.
- Add 8 cups water, vegetables, and seasonings to pot, and bring to a boil.
- Reduce heat to low, and simmer 2 hours or until beans are tender and soup has thickened slightly.
- Stir in pasta and cook until pasta is tender.

Makes 8 servings

Nutrition Facts

Per serving (1 cup): 174 calories, 0 g fat, 10 g protein, 32 g carbohydrates, 7 g fiber, 336 mg sodium

BRAN MUFFINS WITH TANGY ORANGE GLAZE

A high-fiber diet can help control weight, lower cholesterol levels, and possibly lower the risk for colon cancer. Good sources of fiber include fruits, vegetables, whole grain breads and cereals, and dried beans.

Ingredients

Muffin

- 1 cup high-fiber dry cereal, such as All Bran® or Fiber One®
- ⅔ cup orange juice
- ⅓ cup honey
- 2 tablespoons canola oil
- 1 egg

- 1½ cups dry baking mix, such as Bisquick®
- ½ teaspoon baking soda
- ½ cup toasted sunflower seeds, chopped almonds, or chopped walnuts

Orange glaze: Mix the following

- ½ cup powdered sugar
- 2–3 teaspoons orange juice
- ½ teaspoon grated orange peel

Directions

- Preheat oven to 400°F. Line a muffin pan with paper or foil liners.
- Crush cereal in a food processor or by placing in a plastic bag and rolling with a rolling pin. Set aside.
- In a small bowl, mix orange juice, honey, oil, and egg. Set aside.
- Mix baking mix, cereal, baking soda, and half of the nuts (¼ cup) in a medium bowl.
- Stir in the orange juice mixture, stirring just until moistened.
- Divide batter evenly into muffin cups. Sprinkle with remainder of nuts or seeds.
- Bake for 20 minutes or until golden brown.
- Remove from pan. Cool 5 minutes, and drizzle with orange glaze.

Makes 12 servings

Nutrition Facts

Per serving (1 muffin): 190 calories, 8 g fat, 4 g protein, 29 g carbohydrates, 3 g fiber, 350 mg sodium

QUINOA PRIMAVERA

Quinoa, pronounced "keen-wa," is a high-protein grain with a sweet, nutty flavor. This delicious dish provides adequate protein and is full of vegetables to provide plenty of antioxidants in your diet!

Ingredients

1½ cups uncooked quinoa
3 cups chicken broth
3 oz low-fat cream cheese
1 tablespoon chopped fresh basil
1 tablespoon olive oil
2 cloves garlic, chopped

5 cups thinly sliced or chopped vegetables (such as asparagus, broccoli, peppers, carrots, or zucchini)
Grated Romano or Parmesan cheese for garnish

Directions

- Rinse quinoa thoroughly and drain.
- Heat quinoa and broth to boiling in a 2-quart saucepan.
- Reduce heat, cover, and simmer 15 minutes or until quinoa has absorbed the broth.
- Stir in the cream cheese and basil.
- Heat olive oil in a skillet over medium heat and add garlic, stirring just until golden.
- Add vegetables and stir frequently, about 2–3 minutes until vegetables are crisp-tender.
- Toss vegetables and quinoa mixture, and sprinkle with grated cheese.

Makes 6 servings

Nutrition Facts

Per serving: 240 calories, 5 g fat, 12 g protein, 37 g carbohydrates, 5 g fiber, 610 mg sodium

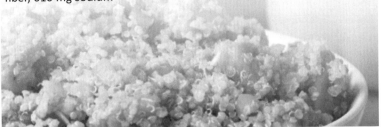

VEGETABLE DIP

Break free from the traditional sour cream–based dips for your veggies. This dip is made with roasted vegetables and is blended to a creamy texture—making it the perfect match for your dipping vegetables. And it's packed full of phytochemicals and antioxidants to keep you healthy!

Ingredients

2 cups sliced zucchini

2 cups sliced yellow summer squash

1 red pepper, sliced

1 red onion, thinly sliced

2 cloves garlic, peeled

¼ teaspoon cayenne pepper

¼ teaspoon salt (optional)

Directions

- Preheat oven to 400°F.
- Spread vegetables on a baking sheet, and spray with nonstick cooking spray.
- Sprinkle with cayenne pepper and salt, if desired.
- Bake about 30 minutes, or until vegetables are tender and lightly browned, turning vegetables often.
- Remove from oven, and place vegetables in a food processor or blender. Cover and blend on high speed until smooth.
- Serve warm, or refrigerate and serve cold with your favorite vegetables for dipping like carrots, peppers, celery, broccoli, and cauliflower. You can even spread on crackers or pita chips for a healthy snack!

Makes 8 servings

Nutrition Facts

Per serving (¼ cup): 20 calories, 0 g fat, 1 g protein, 5 g carbohydrates, 1 g fiber, 150 mg sodium

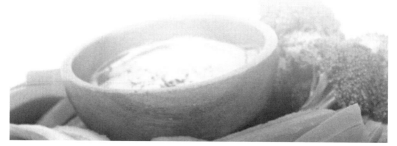

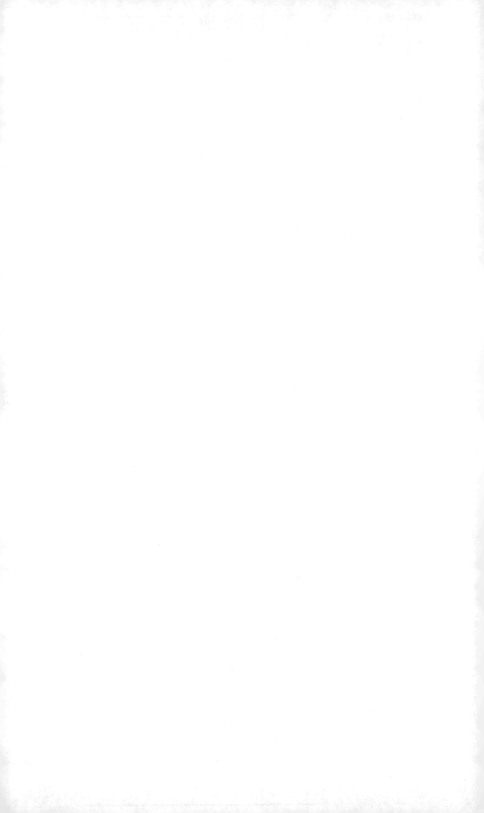

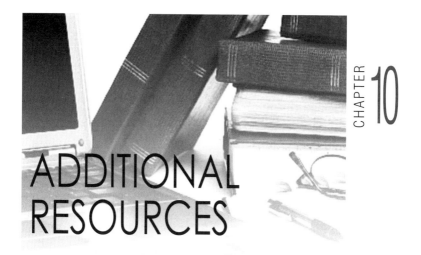

CHAPTER 10

ADDITIONAL RESOURCES

American Cancer Society

*Information on cancer, treatment, services available, and
   survivorship*

800-ACS-2345

www.cancer.org

American Dietetic Association

*Organization of food and nutrition professionals; provides
   general, current nutrition information*

800-877-1600

www.eatright.org

American Institute for Cancer Research

Information specific to nutrition, diet, and cancer

800-843-8114

www.aicr.org

Cancer*Care*

*Patient advocacy program with focus on providing
   education and support for patients with cancer and their
   families*

800-913-HOPE

www.cancercare.org

Cancer Dietitian

Lifestyle tips for prevention and survivorship. Registered dietitian Julie Lanford, MPH, RD, CSO, LDN, offers her expertise to others via her blog and Web site.

www.cancerdietitian.com

Cancer Services

A local, independent nonprofit organization located in Baton Rouge, Louisiana, dedicated to improving life for those living with cancer. The goal is to fill the gaps during and after a cancer diagnosis.

225-927-2273

www.cancerservices.org

Cancer Survivors Network

Information related to surviving and thriving after cancer; sponsored by the American Cancer Society

www.acscsn.org

Caring4Cancer

An online source of knowledge and support for people with cancer; provides information specific to nutrition, diet, and cancer

www.caring4cancer.com

Chemo Care

Information on chemotherapy medications and symptom management during chemotherapy; sponsored by the Scott Hamilton CARES (Cancer Alliance for Research, Education and Survivorship) Initiative at the Cleveland Clinic Taussig Cancer Center

www.chemocare.com

ConsumerLab

Watchdog organization with information on nutritional supplements, warnings, and recalls; fee required for full site access

www.consumerlab.com

A Dietitian's Cancer Story
*Written by registered dietitian and three-time cancer
survivor Diana Dyer, this site provides information
regarding nutrition and cancer survivorship.*
www.cancerrd.com

National Cancer Institute
*Information on clinical trials, nutrition during cancer
treatments and beyond, and supportive care*
800-4-CANCER
www.nci.nih.gov/cancertopics

**National Center for Complementary and
Alternative Medicine**
*Objective information on complementary and alternative
medicines and products*
888-644-6226
www.nccam.nih.gov

Office of Dietary Supplements
*Health information on all types of dietary supplements from
the National Institutes of Health*
301-435-2920
www.ods.od.nih.gov

OncoLink
*Comprehensive cancer information from the Abramson
Cancer Center of the University of Pennsylvania for
patients and their families*
www.oncolink.com

Oncology Nursing Society
*A professional organization of registered nurses and other
healthcare providers dedicated to excellence in patient
care, education, research, and administration in oncology
nursing*
www.ons.org

Oncology Nutrition Dietetic Practice Group

A specialty subgroup of the American Dietetic Association composed of dietitians who work in the oncology field; Web site provides information on oncology nutrition, research, prevention, teatment, and palliative care.

www.oncologynutrition.org

Susan G. Komen for the Cure

Patient education and support for breast cancer survivors; Web site provides information on diet and nutrition.

877-GO-KOMEN

www.komen.org

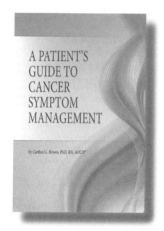
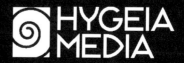

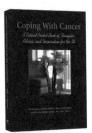
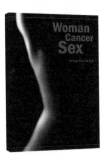
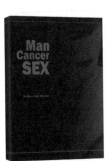
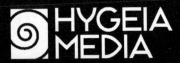